Nursing Student Success

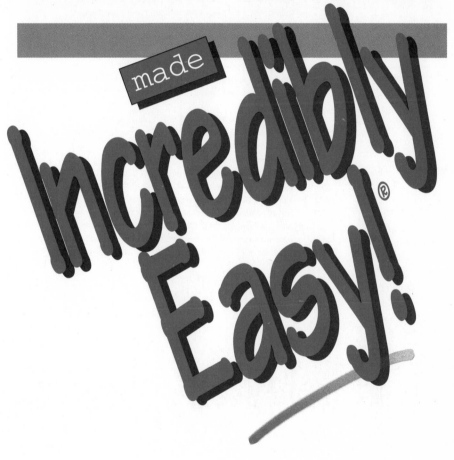

made **Incredibly Easy!**®

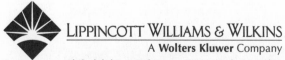

LIPPINCOTT WILLIAMS & WILKINS
A **Wolters Kluwer** Company

Philadelphia • Baltimore • New York • London
Buenos Aires • Hong Kong • Sydney • Tokyo

Staff

Executive Publisher
Judith A. Schilling McCann, RN, MSN

Editorial Director
David Moreau

Clinical Director
Joan M. Robinson, RN, MSN

Senior Art Director
Arlene Putterman

Art Director
Mary Ludwicki

Editorial Project Manager
Tracy S. Diehl

Clinical Project Manager
Tamara Kear, RN, MSN, CNN

Editors
Laura Bruck, Brenna H. Mayer

Clinical Editors
Marcy Caplin, RN, MSN;
Roseanne Hanlon Rafter, RN, MSN, CS

Copy Editors
Kimberly Bilotta (supervisor), Scotti Cohn,
Shana Harrington, Pamela Wingrod

Designer
Lynn Foulk

Illustrator
Bot Roda

Digital Composition Services
Diane Paluba (manager), Joyce Rossi Biletz

Manufacturing
Patricia K. Dorshaw (director), Beth J. Welsh

Editorial Assistants
Megan L. Aldinger, Karen J. Kirk, Linda K. Ruhf

Indexer
Karen C. Comerford

Library of Congress Cataloging-in-Publication Data

Nursing student success made incredibly easy.
    p. ; cm.
Includes index.
1. Nursing students. 2. Nursing schools.
3. Nursing — Study and teaching. I. Lippincott
Williams & Wilkins.
[DNLM: 1. Students, Nursing. 2. Education,
Nursing. WY 18 N9857 2005]

RT73.N825 2005
610.73'071'1 — dc22
ISBN13: 978-1-58255-369-6
ISBN10: 1-58255-369-6 (alk. paper)   2004026611

Contents

Advisory board

Contributors and consultants

Marguerite Ambrose, DNSc, APRN,BC
Assistant Professor
Immaculata (Pa.) University

Janice S. DuBrueler, DNSc(c), RN
Assistant Professor of Nursing
Shenandoah University
Winchester, Va.

Shelba Durston, RN, MSN, CCRN
Nursing Instructor
San Joaquin Delta College
Stockton, Calif.
Staff Nurse
San Joaquin General Hospital
French Camp, Calif.

Karla Jones, RN, MS
Nursing Faculty
Treasure Valley Community College
Ontario, Ore.

Virginia Lester, RN, BSN, MSN
Assistant Professor
Angelo State University
San Angelo, Tex.

Cecilia Jane Maier, RN, MS, CCRN
Assistant Professor
Mount Carmel College of Nursing
Columbus, Ohio

Carolyn H. Mason, RN, MS
Assistant Professor of Nursing
Miami University
Middletown, Ohio

Monica Narvaez Ramirez, RN, MSN
Nursing Instructor
University of the Incarnate Word
School of Nursing and Health Professions
San Antonio, Tex.

Foreword

How exciting that you've decided to embark on a nursing career! When I entered my nursing program, I was elated—and a little afraid.

Becoming a nurse can feel daunting at times. There's a great deal of information to remember, organize, and synthesize. I remember wishing for a resource that would provide me with information on developing good study habits, test-taking strategies, time management skills, and, most importantly, ways to review and prepare for the NCLEX® exam. Unfortunately, during my nursing school experience, there weren't many resources written for the student nurse.

With that in mind, I'm thrilled that this exceptional resource is available to you. *Nursing Student Success Made Incredibly Easy* is informative, easy-to-read, and conveniently organized to provide you with the tools you need to be a successful nursing student.

It also features icons that make learning fun:

Advice from the experts—presents tips for nursing students from professionals.

Exercise your mind—outlines activities to improve study techniques and test-taking skills.

Overcoming obstacles—provides answers to students' difficult questions about studying and test-taking.

No matter what the endeavor, being motivated and focused is essential for success. The first chapter explains the importance of developing a positive attitude and establishing realistic goals. Subsequent chapters deal with such topics as concentration and memory, time management, reading skills, classroom survival skills, test-taking strategies, stress management, clinical labs orientation, and key aspects of planning patient care.

Chapters 9 and 10 are devoted to helping you pass your licensing exam. This section outlines how the exam is organized, how to prepare for the exam, strategies for answering exam questions, prioritizing care using Maslow's hierarchy, and ways to maintain your concentration during the exam.

The last chapter addresses what happens after you pass the exam. All nurses fresh out of nursing school have doubts about whether they're prepared enough to enter into practice. This chapter offers advice on how to be successful as a new graduate, how to search for a job, how to transition into your new role, and how to further develop as a nurse.

I encourage you to take advantage of the tips and strategies this book offers. Being a nursing student isn't easy, but *Nursing Student Success Made Incredibly Easy* can make it less stressful and less overwhelming.

Good luck to you!

Vincent Salyers, RN, EdD
Assistant Professor
University of San Diego
Hahn School of Nursing

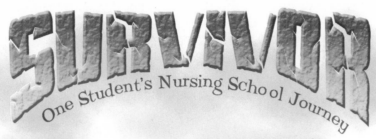

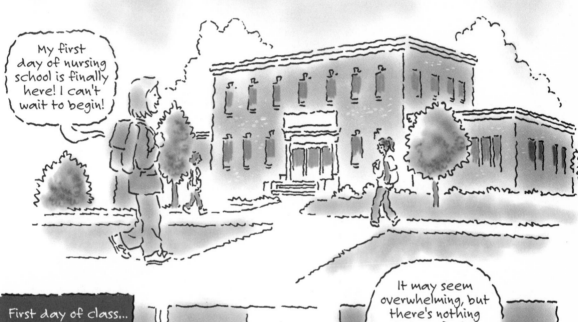

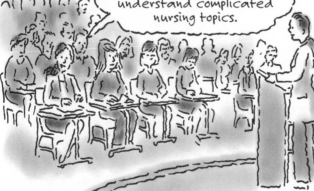

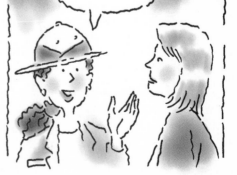

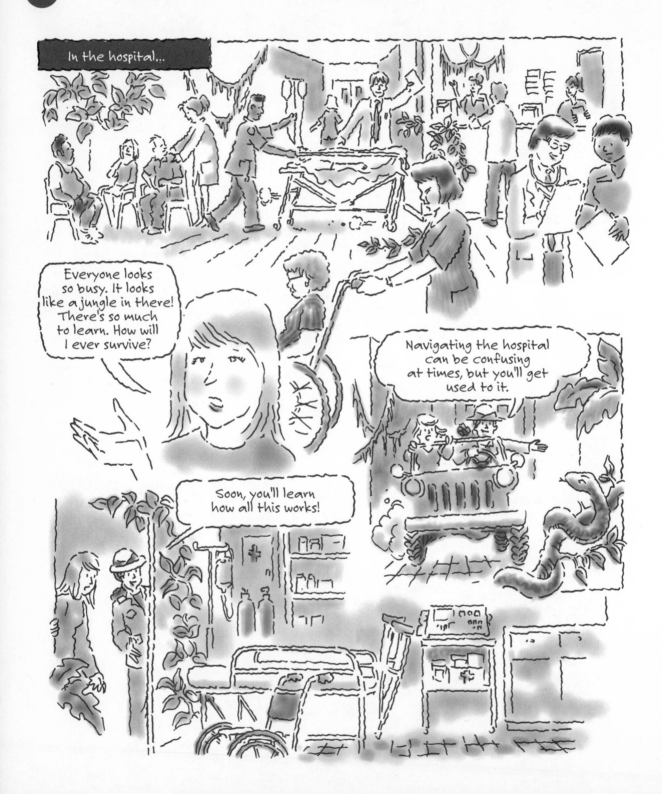

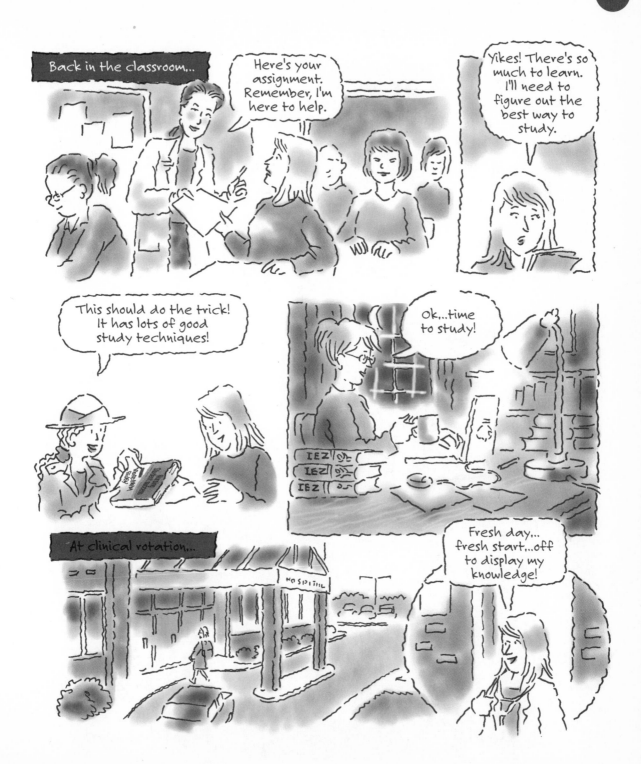

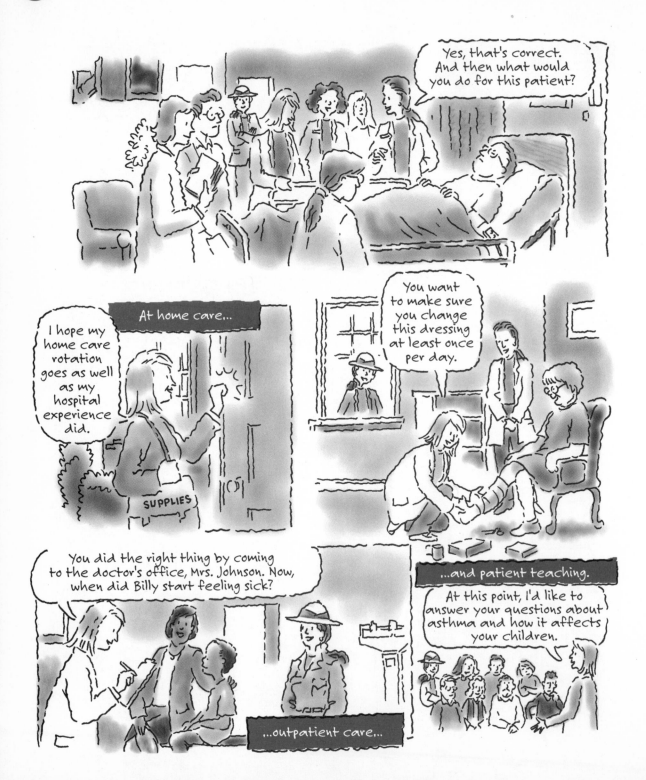

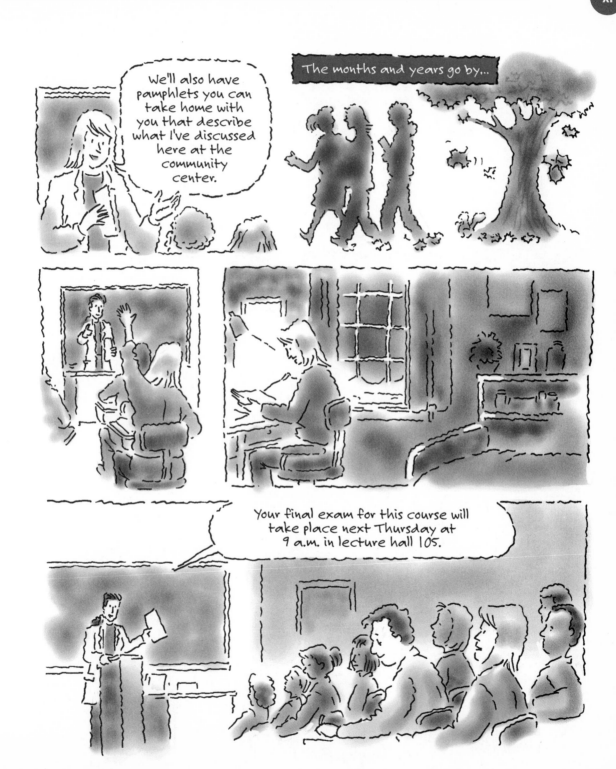

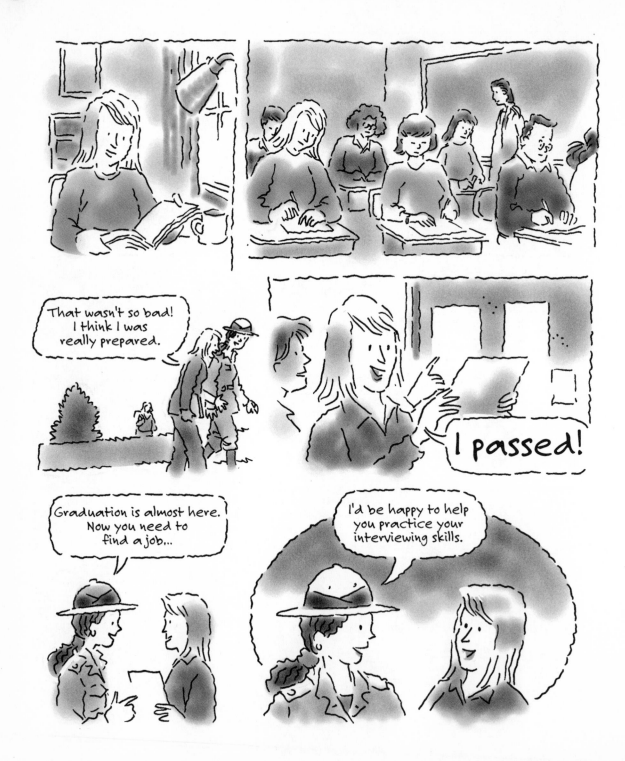

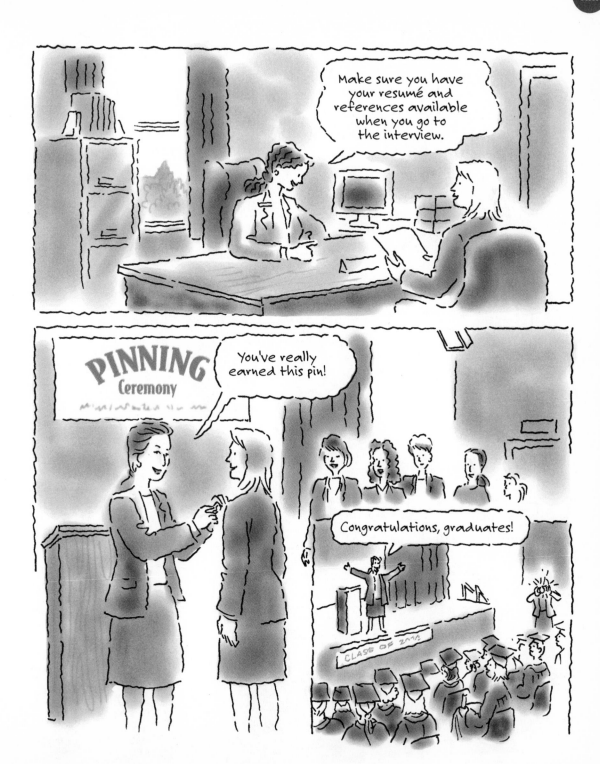

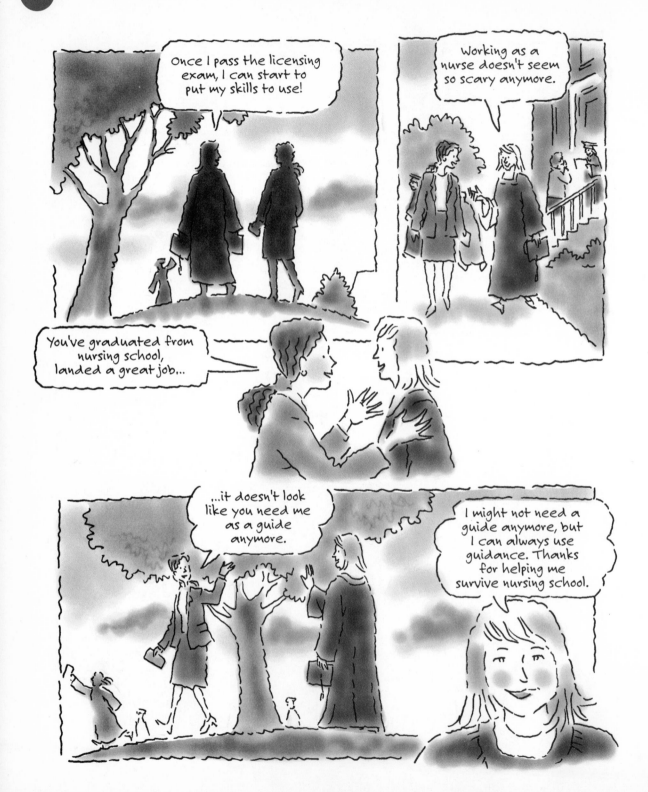

Part I Learning

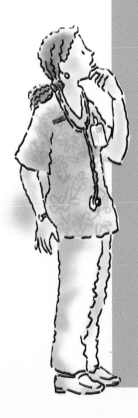

Your attitude and goals

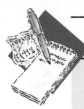

Just the facts

In this chapter, you'll learn:

♦ how a positive, responsible approach to a studying task improves learning

♦ how motivation can be intrinsic (derived from personal desire) or extrinsic (derived from physical reward)

♦ why goals are more likely to be achieved when they're personal rather than set by others

♦ why goals should be specific and have a completion date.

Attitude

Attitude is the approach you take to complete a task. It's often a reflection of how much interest you have in a task or how meaningful the task is to you. Your attitude toward learning, studying, and test taking affects the goals you set for yourself and the techniques and strategies you use to reach those goals. Attitude also strongly affects your level of success in improving your learning skills.

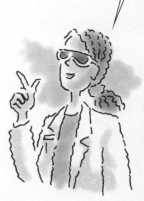

The right attitude can go a long way!

How attitude affects studying

When you approach a difficult subject with the right attitude, you can:

• gain a clear idea of your role in learning
• establish clear learning goals
• study more efficiently
• achieve better grades and improve academic performance.

Attitude meter

Each of the statements below describes someone with a positive attitude. How many of the traits do *you* have?

• You're naturally good at studying.

• You're strongly interested in learning, regardless of the topic.

• You're receptive to new information.

• You don't rely strictly on a teacher to tell you what to study.

• You have faith in yourself and your ability to learn.

• You use a support system as often as possible.

• You take care of your mind and body.

• You keep a consistently positive attitude.

It's up to you

Having the right attitude can be described as having a willingness and desire to learn. Here are some attributes of the "right stuff."

• The student accepts responsibility for learning rather than expecting others to teach her.

• The student participates in the learning process rather than being a passive recipient of knowledge.

• The student actively listens, asks questions, and seeks answers to those questions.

• The student takes charge of what will be learned from the course and, in effect, how well she'll do in the course.

Got it?

How do you know if you have the right attitude about studying? Find out more about your own attitude by checking the "attitude meter." (See *Attitude meter.*)

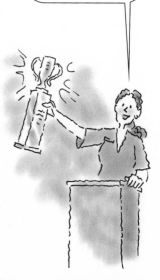

I'd like to thank my colleagues, fellow students, friends, teachers…

Developing a winning attitude

A student with a winning attitude expects success, even when tackling the most complex new material. Such students have faith in their own abilities, particularly in their ability to attend classes, complete assigned readings, conduct research, and understand the material presented. Building and using support systems, taking care of yourself, and maintaining consistent focus on your goals are key to having and keeping a winning attitude.

A little help, please

One way to build and maintain a winning attitude is to seek out and accept support from other people and resources, including:
- colleagues
- fellow students
- formal and informal discussion groups
- friends and family
- resource centers, such as libraries and media centers
- teachers and tutors.

Exercise your attitude

Attitude is often reflected in how well a person takes care of herself. Getting enough sleep, eating properly, and exercising can help maintain a healthy mind, body, and attitude. Looking good and feeling good are big attitude boosters.

Steady as she goes

It's important to keep a positive attitude for the long haul rather than backsliding into complacency in the middle of a task. Developing a good attitude may take time, but it's worth the effort. A consistently positive attitude allows you to cope effectively in the face of minor setbacks, and even major disasters.

Motivation

Motivation is the carrot on a stick that inspires the proverbial mule to move forward. It's the thing that makes a person *want* to do something. Motivation:
- causes a person to initiate an activity. In the case of studying, the motivation may be the need for achievement, a high test score, or a good grade in the course.
- helps the person move toward a goal, closing the gap between the starting point and the final objective.
- spurs the person to persist in her attempts to reach the goal until she succeeds.

Motivation is the carrot on a stick — or the ice cream in the cone — that inspires you to move forward and want to succeed (or eat)!

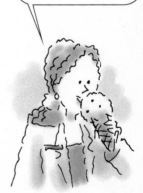

How motivation affects studying

Motivation to improve study skills and succeed at learning may be *intrinsic* (an inborn factor that drives a person to learn) or *extrinsic* (a benefit derived from learning).

Coming from within...

Intrinsic motivation includes:
- a general desire to learn

- a sense of curiosity
- a willingness to take risks
- an innate sense of wanting to excel at something
- an inherent interest in the subject at hand.

...Or without

Extrinsic motivation includes the desire for:
- better grades or test scores
- improved self-esteem
- a sense of fulfillment
- increased competence in the subject being studied
- valuable credentials on a resume
- a better job
- an opportunity to earn a higher salary.

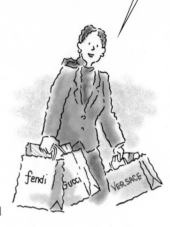

Toward a gold star

Think back to when you were in elementary school. At that time, the reward you received for a job well done may have been a gold star. The teacher's idea was to establish that sticker as a motivator, something you would value and strive to earn.

Adults can establish their own sources of motivation. At the start of a task, decide what your reward will be for your hard work. You may decide that the work itself is its own reward, but you may find it more inspiring to aim for something more — a pat on the back, lunch out with friends, new shoes, or a few days of rest and relaxation.

Reach for the sky

When choosing a motivator, aim high. Choose a motivator that makes the hard work worthwhile. Then be sure to collect the reward.

Don't underestimate the value of intangible rewards. You may find that reveling in a sense of satisfaction or accomplishment may be a stronger motivator than earning a more tangible reward.

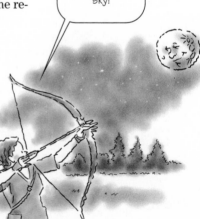

Get personal

To gain insight into personal motivators, think about things you do on a regular basis and then determine the source of motivation for completing each task. For example, suppose you exercise at a gym twice per week. Why do you do that? To look and feel good? To get your dollar's worth of membership dues? To meet new people?

Identifying and understanding your particular motivating factors for non-school-related situations can help you successfully find motivating factors for school-related situations.

Long-lasting rewards

A wide range of long-lasting rewards can be gained from developing successful study habits and improving your test-taking skills. Those rewards include:
• a deeper understanding of the subject matter
• an ability to apply improved skills to other subject areas
• enhanced self-esteem, leading to greater success in other areas of endeavor
• improved grades and test scores
• improved socioeconomic status as a result of learning marketable skills.

Setting goals

Procrastination, poor concentration, and lack of motivation take root when a student lacks clear goals. Without clearly defined goals, it's easy to become distracted. To avoid distraction, set goals for yourself.

Some goals should be easy to reach and some should be hard. Some goals should be long-term and some short-term. The more attractive the goal, the more motivated you'll be. The goal should be specific and include a time for completion. Setting a time or date for completion of the goal helps you to focus on the goal and gives your day-to-day tasks a sense of purpose.

Don't let procrastination and lack of motivation take root. Setting clearly defined goals will set you free to learn and succeed!

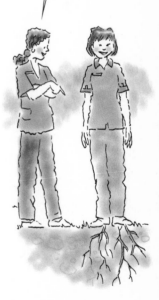

Accomplishing a goal

Accomplishing a goal involves creating a measurable and achievable goal, determining that the goal is something worth working toward, and devising strategies to achieve the goal. These same steps are necessary to formulate a client goal in the nursing process.

Does it measure up?

A goal should be stated in measurable terms. For example, "I want to master the double-entry system of note-taking by the end of October" is a more specific objective than "I want to improve my study skills."

We have the technology

Determine whether the goal is achievable. Is there enough time to pursue the goal and, more important, do you have the necessary skills, strengths, and resources to achieve the goal? If not, modify the goal to make it achievable.

Exercise your mind

Accomplishing a short-term goal

Short-term goals can be accomplished by following a series of steps that gradually move you toward your goal. To accomplish a short-term goal:

• Write the goal in measurable terms.

• Set a date for completing the goal.

• Check that the goal is achievable in the time allotted.

• Identify potential problems and determine ways of preventing them.

• Create a series of specific steps for achieving the goal.

• Set a schedule for completing each step.

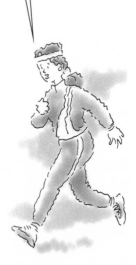

Make your goals desirable and achievable.

Do the ends justify the means?

Make certain that achieving the goal is genuinely desirable and worthwhile. The goal should have a positive impact on your life and be consistent with your most important basic values.

In addition, determine why the goal is worthwhile. Make sure that reaching the goal will give you a sense of accomplishment.

Expect the worst, achieve the best

Anticipate potential problems in meeting your goal. In your mind, take yourself step by step through your plan for achieving the goal and ask yourself what can go wrong at each step. Then plan ways to prevent or overcome these problems.

At the same time, devise strategies and steps for achieving the goal. What will you need to begin? What comes next? Then set a timeline for accomplishing each step. (See *Accomplishing a short-term goal.*)

Goal structures

Students in a classroom can be greatly influenced by other people involved in accomplishing the same goal. The influence of others on your goals has been called the *goal structure* of the task. The three goal structures that have been identified are:

☝ cooperative, in which students believe their goal is attainable only if other students will also reach the same goal

✌ competitive, in which students believe they will reach their goal only if other students don't

individualistic, in which students believe their own attempt to reach a goal isn't related to other students' attempts to reach goals.

Grades and goals

If an instructor concentrates class efforts on competitive grading, students tend to focus on performance goals rather than learning goals. Do as much as you can to focus on learning rather than focusing on getting a good grade or doing the work just to get it finished. By understanding the value of the assigned work and how the information you gain will be useful in the future, you can more readily prepare for learning and, thus, become more successful.

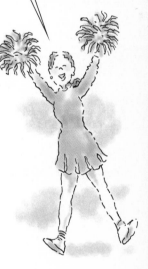

To succeed, you must truly want to succeed. Go for it!

The power of the "A"

Focusing on learning doesn't mean, however, that you shouldn't consider grades at all. Grades are an integral part of the entire school experience and can be powerful motivators themselves. Grades also serve as checkpoints to help you evaluate your progress and adjust your plan for success accordingly. Try to use the desire to earn good grades as a short-term goal without sacrificing the more important long-term goal of getting a good education.

Personal payload

When you're forced to do something you don't really want to do, you'll be less likely to succeed because the goal isn't your own. The successful student must *want* to succeed, and learning itself should be a primary goal and its own reward.

Reaching your goals

Approach each goal you've set for yourself consistently and with a clear sense of purpose. Reaching your goals involves setting goals continually, monitoring your progress, determining time frames for your goals, prioritizing goals, challenging yourself to reach higher goals, committing to success, revising your goals when necessary, and linking short-term goals with longer-term ones.

Getting into the goal-setting habit

If you haven't already begun to set goals, start the habit now. If the goals you've identified so far haven't motivated you as well as you had hoped they would, review the goals and, if necessary, set new ones.

Putting pen to paper

Keep a journal for long-term, intermediate, and short-term goals. Use to-do lists to keep track of the immediate goals that form a part of everyday life. You'll tend to commit your resources more readily to a written goal than to one you've only thought about but haven't recorded. In addition, writing the goal makes it more concrete and easier to review periodically.

List goals according to how long it will take to reach them. Typical goal categories are long-term (5 to 10 years), intermediate (3 to 5 years), short-term (6 months to 2 years), and immediate (this month, this week, or today). Prioritize your goals. Without priorities, you may spend your energy trying to achieve too many goals at once.

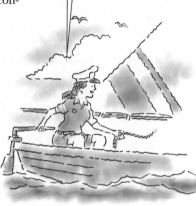

Goal setting is only a tool. Be sure to enjoy your journey and every success along the way.

Challenge yourself

Keep your goals high enough to inspire you and reasonable enough to seem always within your reach. For example, if your long-term goal is to be a registered nurse, your intermediate goal may be to finish nursing school. You may find that your greatest challenge lies in becoming one of the top students in your class.

Commit to the actions required to achieve the goal. Understand that you may not succeed immediately. Learn from your failures and reassess your action plan.

Rewrite, revise, revisit, review

Review your goals and revise them as necessary. At certain points, more inspiring goals may present themselves and short-term and immediate goals may require revision. It's better to change goals and strategies as circumstances change than to lose focus on your long-term goals by refusing to change short-term ones.

The domino effect

Long-term, intermediate, short-term, and immediate goals should be linked in focus to your overriding goals. For example, reading 15 pages of course material today (your immediate goal) leads to achieving a good grade in the class (short-term goal), which leads to graduation from nursing school (intermediate goal), which, in turn, leads to the opportunity to become a registered nurse (long-term goal).

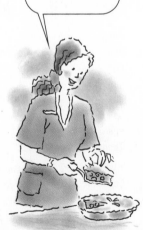

Slicing larger goals into smaller pieces makes big tasks more palatable.

Types of goals

Long-term study goals generally relate to career goals. However, some people simply enjoy studying as a means of self-improvement. Again, if the long-term goal is truly the student's choice, then the student is self-motivated and excited about the result, prompting the student to keep studies on track. Like a basketball player who keeps a photo of Michael Jordan on the refrigerator, having some tangible reminder of the rewards of that long-term goal is useful.

Intermediate goals are usually 3 to 5 years in the future and are keys to achieving long-term goals. For example, careers that require extended education necessitate the intermediate goal of acceptance into the appropriate centers for higher learning.

Hops, skips, and jumps

The steps toward an intermediate goal are a series of *short-term goals,* usually set 6 months to 2 years in the future. Particularly when studying toward a goal (such as a certain degree), the short-term goals could be set per semester or per academic year.

The dash

Each short-term goal can be further divided into smaller tasks, or *immediate goals,* which can be accomplished in 30 minutes to an hour on a daily basis until each study task is completed. A series of 15 to 20 small tasks might be part of the plan for completing an otherwise frustrating 20-page paper. The result is a finished essay and the chance to experience 15 to 20 successes along the way! (See *Accomplishing a long-term goal.*)

Memory jogger

Setting goals is an invitation to success. As with any invitation, you should *RSVP.* Make your goals reasonable, specific, verifiable, and with a payoff at the end.

Exercise your mind

Accomplishing a long-term goal

Although long-term goals can be daunting to think about, keeping an eye focused on them can help you accomplish short-term goals more successfully. To accomplish a long-term goal, begin by describing where you want to be in 20 years. What do you want to be doing, and where? Write down these 20-year goals. Then ask yourself these questions:

• What will I need to accomplish in 5 years to be able to reach my 20-year goal? (Write down these goals as your 5-year goals.)

• What will I need to accomplish in 6 months to be able to reach each 5-year goal? (Write down these goals as your 6-month goals.)

• What will I need to accomplish this week to reach my 6-month goals? (Write down these goals as your weekly goals.)

Examine the goals

Now list at least five reasons it's important for you to reach your 20-year goal. List at least three negative things that could happen if you don't reach your goal.

Oh, what to do, what to do?

When immediate goals are listed and prioritized, a daily to-do list is created. Each goal must:
- be reasonable (can be completed in 30 to 60 minutes)
- be specific
- be verifiable or measurable (can be crossed off the list when it's completed)
- have a payoff (reward) when achieved.

Treats for triumph

Rewards give you additional reasons to reach a goal. A reward can be small or large, depending on the person and the goal. To serve as an effective motivator, a reward should be desirable. You might reward yourself with dinner at your favorite restaurant or that CD you've had your eye on for the last few weeks.

The reward should also fit the task. That means finishing a task that takes all of 30 minutes doesn't necessarily warrant a weekend shopping trip.

Peers and punishment

In addition to rewards, other types of external motivation include peer pressure and punishment. By sharing goals with a friend, you create additional pressure to perform. Punishment, when you deny yourself certain privileges if you don't complete a task, rarely works as a motivator.

Missing the mark

If you fall short of a short-term goal, you may become discouraged and miss a step toward achieving a long-term goal. Try to recoup the loss by reviewing your goals and adjusting them and their deadlines as appropriate. In the long run, it's more efficient to achieve the goal in the first place, even if it's a little behind schedule. (See *Evaluating a goal.*)

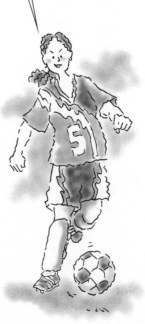

If you miss your goal, try to remain upbeat. Review your goal, and adjust as necessary.

Staying on task

Sometimes it's hard to get started on a project or assignment. The important thing is to take some action, even if it's not as much as you had planned. To get yourself started, break a large project down into manageable parts, and then schedule deadlines for completing each part. Gaining closure on each part, handling deadlines effectively, avoiding *burnout* (a state of exhaustion and loss of motivation), and juggling all your other responsibilities efficiently will keep you on the right path toward your goals.

Exercise your mind

Evaluating a goal

Evaluating a goal is a different process than creating one. Evaluation allows you to create more useful, achievable goals. Practice evaluating a goal by completing this exercise. Decide whether each of the listed goals is satisfactory or if it's lacking in some way. Use the key to denote your decision. Keep in mind that if a goal is unsatisfactory, more than one letter may apply.

Key

S— Satisfactory

M—Measurable outcomes lacking

D— Deadline lacking

O— Other people are needed to achieve the goal

Goals

1. _____ Define my success in each clinical rotation by my score on the care plan.

2. _____ Know all assigned mathematical formulas by the end of next month.

3. _____ Appreciate art more fully as the result of visiting an art gallery.

4. _____ By Tuesday, identify the handouts to be used for the final examination.

5. _____ Learn more about genetic engineering.

6. _____ Become a better reader.

7. _____ Improve my anatomy and physiology grade by 1 quality point by participating in a group-study project before the end of the term.

8. _____ Complete all assigned medical-surgical readings by next Wednesday.

9. _____ Read my notes immediately after each nutrition class so I can make additions or corrections.

10. _____ Improve my grade in fundamentals by 10 points between the midterm examination and the final examination by joining a study group and meeting with the group 3 days per week for the rest of the marking period.

Your goals

List five of your own goals, and evaluate them.

1._____

2._____

3._____

4._____

5._____

From start to finish

Closure is the positive feeling you get when you finish a task. One way to obtain closure is to divide a task into manageable goals, list them, and check them off the list as each one is finished. For example, to complete a reading assignment on time, divide the total assignment into smaller assignments by setting a certain number of pages as a goal to be reached each day. Every time you reach one of these small goals, you'll feel a sense of closure that will help propel you toward the next goal.

Dueling deadlines

Several tasks might have the same deadline. Although changing from one task to another may give you a break, changing tasks too often actually wastes time. It slows your momentum on one task and necessitates that you'll have to review tasks that have been put aside when you return to them.

To avoid problems from changing tasks too often, determine how much time you have for the task. If you have only an hour, don't switch tasks; an hour isn't enough time to maintain peak efficiency.

When working on a long-term project that needs to be set aside to complete more immediate tasks, stay organized. To ease the return to the first project, make a list of questions, write notes, identify objectives, and compile references, papers, and other materials pertinent to the task. Then keep all the materials in one place so you can reach them easily and get started more quickly.

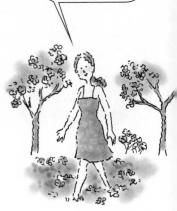

Make sure you take time out for fitness and play...or just taking a stroll.

The juggling act

Everyone has to manage a wide assortment of life activities: fitness, relationships, chores, finances, hobbies, sports, work, and others. Add academics and school activities into the mix, and the need for organization becomes clear. Set aside time each day for work as well as for play to make the most of your time.

When you face what seems like too many tasks to complete at once, prioritize each task by writing the tasks on paper and then assigning each with a 1, 2, or 3, with 1 being the most important tasks and 3 being those that can wait. Then concentrate on completing the 1s, then the 2s, and lastly the 3s. Prioritizing tasks on paper helps you focus on the most important tasks and gives you a sense of accomplishment that you're moving ahead — even if you haven't finished all assigned tasks.

Believe in yourself!

Tell yourself that you can do this: you can pass this course; you can be a nurse. Think about "the little engine that could" in the popular children's book. The engine kept repeating, "I think I can,

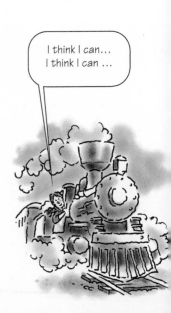

I think I can... I think I can ...

I know I can." Keep telling yourself that you *can* do it. With hard work and organization, you can accomplish your goals.

You have chosen to undertake a profession with difficult and changing subject matter. If nursing were easy, there would never be a nursing shortage. At the first sign of problems, seek help. Most faculty will give help to a struggling student who has motivation, desire, and a good attitude, and who works to accomplish goals. Asking for help is a sign of strength, not weakness.

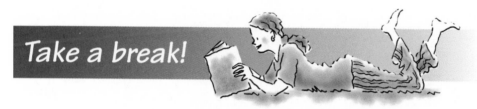

At a crossroads

Look for key terms in the crossword puzzle below. Relax and enjoy — don't stress! (Answer key on next page.)

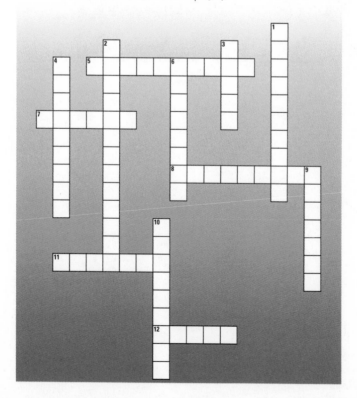

Across

5. Incentive to perform a task

7. Marks indicating quality of work

8. Due dates

11. State of exhaustion from overwork

12. To consider in detail

Down

1. A pledge

2. Focus

3. Objectives

4. An inborn motivational factor

6. State of mind; approach

9. Favorable outcome

10. A motivational benefit from learning

Answer key

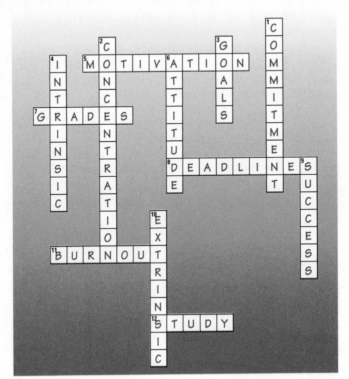

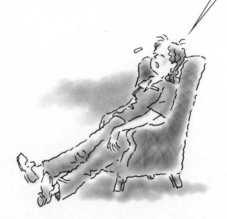

Whew. It's times like this that I could use a relaxing crossword puzzle!

Controlling that meandering mind

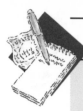

Just the facts

In this chapter, you'll learn:

♦ how important it is to have good concentration

♦ how the brain processes through registration, short-term memory, long-term memory, and working memory

♦ why effective study strategies include practice, spaced study, reduction of interference, associations, lists, and imagery

♦ how memory skills can be improved by using various memory enhancement strategies.

Concentration

The more focused your concentration, the more efficiently you can use your study time. To improve your concentration skills, first identify the distractions that impede concentration. Then use one or more study techniques to improve your ability to concentrate and, thus, to learn.

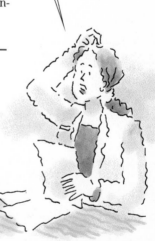

Now, let's see. Daily dosage = ice cream = popcorn...? Wow! Hunger sure can be distracting when you're trying to study!

Distractions

Distractions that interfere with concentration can originate from internal or external sources. An *internal distraction* is something you think or feel that detracts from focusing on your studies. Hunger and emotions, such as anger or sadness, are internal sources of distraction. *External distractions* stem from something in your study environment. Loud noises, an uncomfortable chair, and poor lighting are examples of external sources of distraction.

Advice from the experts

Meandering mind

Some people seem to remember everything they hear and see, including the entire name of a person they've just met. Others find that their minds tend to wander easily and can't remember as much as they'd like. Do you have a meandering mind? To find out how well you tend to pay attention, ask yourself the questions below. The more you answer yes, the more likely it is that you have a meandering mind and could benefit from strategies to improve your concentration.

- Do you generally forget the names of people you just met?
- Do you find yourself commonly asking people to repeat what they've just said?
- Do you tend to lose track of what's going on, as if you're snapping out of a daydream in the middle of an event?
- Do you sometimes stare blankly at a page?
- Do you sometimes feel as if you don't remember what you've just read, even though you know you read the material?

Slow down, you talk too fast!

Sometimes, people — even your instructors — can be sources of external distraction. (See *Meandering mind.*) The instructor may speak rapidly, covering a lot of material in a short time. Conversely, the instructor may speak slowly, causing you to become bored and unable to concentrate fully.

Where's my dictionary?

The instructor may use jargon or big words without clear meanings, either of which makes understanding the material more difficult and impedes your concentration. Regardless of the source, you need to learn how to deal with distractions and to concentrate your attention fully on the material under study.

Learning to concentrate

To improve your concentration skills, you must *want* to learn the material. Internal motivation is the key to initiating and maintaining concentration. In addition, you need to be awake and alert, and prepared to see, hear, and learn. Being awake and alert allows you to use your class or study time more efficiently and removes the need to review the material a second time when it should have been learned the first time.

Improving your concentration during class and study sessions can help improve retention and foster better scores on tests, quizzes, and assignments.

Eyes front

During class time, try these strategies to help you stay focused:
• Sit up front. The closer you sit to the front, the less distraction there will be between you and the instructor.
• Take a walk between classes to calm down. Walk briskly for 5 to 10 minutes to help ease tension.
• Meditate before class. Find a calm place, close your eyes, sit up straight, relax your arms and legs, and picture something simple, still, and peaceful. Breathe deeply and slowly for about 5 minutes.
• Limit caffeine intake. Caffeine is a central nervous system stimulant. Although a little caffeine can heighten awareness temporarily, too much caffeine can make you jumpy and reduce your ability to concentrate.

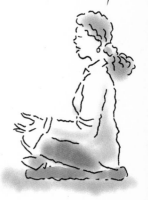

Ohmmm. I'm calm, focused, and ready to take on the world...or at least organic chemistry!

Study hard, study right!

Try these strategies to help improve concentration during study sessions:
• Study when the time is right for you, during periods of alertness.
• Study in a familiar, comfortable place.
• Study under natural light (sunlight) or incandescent light (an ordinary light bulb) rather than fluorescent light, to lessen eye strain.
• Set realistic study goals for a study session.
• Make a specific to-do list before you start studying.
• Focus your study on one topic at a time.
• Drink water to prevent dehydration and enhance your ability to maintain focus.
• Vary your study activities. For instance, include in your study time reading, taking notes, and just plain thinking to keep your study process active.
• Take short breaks in your studying every 45 minutes to 1 hour.
• Remove visual distractions from the study area. These distractions can break concentration and stimulate daydreaming.
• Study in an atmosphere of *white noise*, a low-level background sound that masks outside distractions. For example, the sound of soft instrumental music can help mask the annoying sound of a clattering air conditioner.

Power napping

If you're having trouble staying awake and alert when studying, try taking a power nap. A short nap of 5 to 15 minutes — but not longer — can rejuvenate the body and mind. Research indicates that a power nap can replenish the level of amines in the brain. Amines play a role in helping you maintain attention and remain alert and aware.

Improving concentration

There's nothing like practice to improve your concentration. Strategies for improving concentration skills include maintaining a consistent state of mind, reading and relaxing, and *thinking globally* (within a large framework of knowledge).

Stress-free learning and recall

If you're relaxed during study, you're more likely to recall information better than if you were tired or stressed when you studied. To reduce stress during studying, keep yourself rested and learn to work within a global framework.

Give your brain a break

Ideally, you should rest right before a test and before and right after learning new material. Your brain needs time to relax, sort through information, and then store the information for later retrieval. Sleep is particularly important in this regard. During deep sleep, the brain continues to sort and store information, saving important memories and allowing unnecessary ones to be forgotten.

However, keep in mind that during sleep you can forget important information if your brain hasn't moved it out of short-term memory. Before you go to sleep at night, make a short quiz of 5 to 10 questions from the material you think you've learned. When you wake up in the morning, take the quiz to see how you do. If you've forgotten important information, study it again.

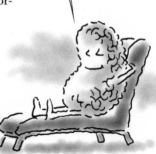

Don't forget to give me a break! I process information better when I'm rested.

Think globally, study locally

The brain is able to recall information more efficiently when the item being recalled exists within a larger framework of knowledge, or more global understanding. For example, a small area of a street map is easier to understand and recall when considered within the larger framework of a map of the entire city.

In applying this concept to studying, try to learn more about a topic in general before focusing on the particular assigned topic. Television programs, videos, or film documentaries can be good sources of such information, as can magazine articles written for the lay public.

For instance, if you've been assigned a topic of caring for a patient after a coronary artery bypass graft, you might start your studying by reading an article on heart surgery in *Newsweek*, *Reader's Digest*, or another lay publication. Then, when you read about coronary artery bypass grafting in a professional textbook, you'll be able to apply the new knowledge more readily and remember key facts longer.

Memory

Information is stored in different ways and in different forms, which is why you can remember some things clearly and others hardly at all. Memory isn't a sense but a skill that can be developed and improved.

Early memories

Most people can't recall the first year of their life. That's because brain structures responsible for memory don't fully develop until about age 2. In addition, children generally learn to speak after their first year of life, not before. As a result, information stored as memories during the first year of life can't be stored in words.

Some events in childhood, though, remain as clear, vivid memories long after the event has taken place in that person's history. For instance, you may clearly remember your first day in school. That's probably because going to school was a new event for you and your brain had to create a new category for it. Later on, going to school became less and less memorable.

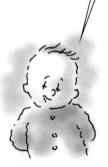

Goo-goo bah poo! I probably won't remember this stuff until I can store information as real words.

Processing information

How your brain processes memories determines what you remember and what you forget. The three basic stages involved in information processing are:

 registration

 short-term memory

 long-term memory. (See *Making memories last*, page 22.)

Registration

In *registration,* the initial stage of information processing, information is received and may eventually be understood and selected to be remembered. The process of registration involves three phases: reception, perception, and selection.

What a lovely reception

In *reception,* you sense something or someone but you don't yet recognize what it is or what it means. For instance, you might auscultate a patient's bowel sounds and hear noises but have no idea what they mean or what condition they represent.

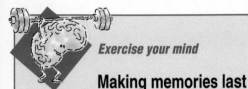

Exercise your mind

Making memories last

There are many ways to embed what you learn in your long-term memory. Putting these tips into your study regimen can help you retain key information.

Working alone

• Attach a strong emotion to the material.

• Rewrite the material.

• Build a working model of a physical aspect of the material being studied.

• Create a song about the material or change the words to an existing song.

• Draw a picture or create a poster using intense colors.

• Repeat and review the material within 10 minutes, 48 hours, and 7 days.

• Smear a droplet of your favorite perfume onto a reminder note to help you remember the contents of the note.

• Summarize the material in your notes.

• Try to immediately apply what you've learned to activities in your daily life.

• Use mnemonics and acronyms to organize the material.

• Write about the material in a journal.

Working with others

• Act out the material or role-play a situation related to the material being studied.

• Join a study group or other support group.

• Discuss the information with a peer to gain an additional perspective and solidify the material in your mind.

• Make a video or audiotape related to the material being studied.

• Make up and tell a story about the material.

At least, that's my perception

In the second phase, *perception*, you recognize what you've seen and attach a meaning to it. For example, when auscultating bowel sounds, you hear a whooshing sound. You've already learned in class that a whooshing sound could represent an obstruction of some kind. When you hear the whooshing, you consider that the patient may have an obstruction of some kind. You've attached a meaning to a sound you recognized: that's perception.

Be selective

The final phase of registration involves *selection*, in which your brain selects information to be remembered. The information selected depends on a number of factors, including the:
- material at hand
- purpose for remembering
- learner's background knowledge
- content and difficulty level of the information
- way the information is organized.

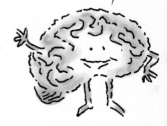

Hmmm, is this something I want to think about and process, or ignore?

Is it useful?

A person selectively ignores or processes information depending on the usefulness of the information in meeting the person's goals. Information perceived by the learner to be useful tends to be processed. Information perceived to be less useful tends to be ignored.

Ignored information is quickly forgotten; processed information is transferred into *short-term memory* — the second stage of memory processing.

Short-term memory

All information selected by the brain to be remembered enters short-term memory, which can last as little as 15 seconds. The brain's short-term memory can't hold much information, nor can it hold the information for long. Research indicates that short-term memory can hold five to nine chunks of information, depending on how well the information is grouped.

For example, the numbers 1, 8, 6, 0, 1, 8, 6, and 4 can be recalled by chunking the numbers into dates — 1860 and 1864. *Chunking* the information into smaller bits makes it easier to recall the information and allows more memory space for other information.

Chunking up info

When learning new information, your brain has more difficulty organizing, or chunking, the new information because it's unsure of the relationships between pieces of information. That's why learning small chunks of material at a time works better than trying to learn one large chunk all at once.

Wait, there's more

Such factors as age, maturation, amount of practice, meaningfulness of the information, and complexity of information also affect the size of short-term memory. From short-term memory, the brain either forgets the information or moves it to long-term memory.

Long-term memory

After you rehearse and chunk information, your brain can move it to long-term memory. Information stored in *long-term memory* is organized and stored for long periods, but its duration there depends on how completely the information has been processed and how often you use it. Although many techniques can be used to aid in the transfer of information from short-term to long-term memory, the most important one is to use the information right away.

Working memory

Researchers have developed the term *working memory* to describe how your brain stores and retrieves information from short-term and long-term memory. You can improve your *working memory* — your ability to store and recall information — through the use of four specific strategies:

 selection

 association

 organization

 rehearsal.

Selection

During *selection*, choose the information you want to remember and begin selecting ways to process the information. For instance, if you need to learn the steps involved in taking a blood pressure, you need to first decide that the information is important. You know that you'll need to recall the steps in the process in actual practice, so you almost unconsciously decide that the material is important.

Being more consciously aware of what material is important is a key first step in learning the information. When you *really* want to know someone's name, you make a conscious effort to remember it. For instance, you may choose to remember a doctor's last name but not his first name because you'll most likely address him as "Doctor", not by his first name. Learning new material begins with making a conscious decision to remember it.

Association

After selecting the information you want to remember, create an *association* to the information. For instance, to remember infor-

What was
his name
again...?
Frank, Bob...

mation about a particular disease, you might associate that material with a patient you once cared for who had the disease. The associations you make between something you already know and something you're trying to learn serve as memory cues that allow you to more easily retrieve the information later.

Organization

During *organization*, memorization takes place in an ordered way. You may decide there are too many steps in taking a blood pressure to memorize all at once, so you break the process into smaller chunks, each consisting of only a few steps. Now that the longer list is made up of several smaller steps, you can push the information into long-term memory through repetition. Rewriting the steps, repeating the steps verbally, or role-playing the steps will help you remember them more efficiently and will clear your working memory for the next piece of new information to be learned. *Mnemonics* — memory aids, such as acronyms, acrostics, associations, and rhymes — can be particularly effective in organizing chunks of information.

Rehearsal

Rehearsal involves repeatedly reviewing information you've learned. Take a tip from the acting profession: One of the best ways to memorize material is to repeat it — or rehearse it — over and over for short periods of time.

Practice makes perfect

These short bursts of rehearsal are more effective than long bouts of rehearsal. For example, rather than rehearsing the steps in taking a blood pressure repeatedly for 1 hour each day, rehearse the steps for 15 minutes four times per day. Frequency of rehearsal really pays off when you have a lot of information to remember.

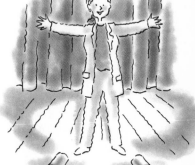

Just like lines in a play, study material is best remembered when you repeat it over and over again. Just like lines in a play, study material is...

Memory retrieval

After information is processed, it may or may not remain in long-term memory. Information that doesn't remain in long-term memory is forgotten. Information may be forgotten as a result of infrequent use, depending on how interested you are in the information, what your purpose is for learning, how frequently you use the information, and how many connections with other pieces of information you've made for the memory.

Exercise your mind

Searching for a lost memory

Can't remember something important? Try these strategies to search for a lost memory.

1. Say or write down everything you can remember that relates to the information you're seeking.

2. Try to recall events or information in a different order.

3. Re-create the learning environment or relive the event. Include sounds, smells, details of weather, nearby objects, other people who were present, what you said or thought at the time, and how you felt.

Interested?

In general, the more interested you are in a topic, the stronger your memory of it will be. For instance, if you know you'll be quizzed on a particular piece of information in anatomy class, you'll be more likely to commit that information to long-term memory. Purpose, frequency of use, and number of connections all play similar roles in forming long-term memories.

Now, where did I put those keys?

The ability to answer questions regarding information you learned a long time ago depends on your ability to recall seldom-used information. Such information may be difficult, or even impossible, to locate in memory because it hasn't been used in a long time. (See *Searching for a lost memory.*)

Up to the challenge?

To keep your long-term memory ready for challenges, plan a review session once each month. During your review, read aloud your notes from the previous month and add bookmarks to your notes so you can find the content easily later. For instance, if you drew a diagram of the bones of the forearm in your notes, put a note in the margin so you can find the corresponding section of your textbook. If you missed a question on a recent test, highlight and rewrite your notes about the question so you'll know the correct answer the next time.

Spending an hour or two each month reviewing information will help keep it fresh in your mind and keep those synapses firing.

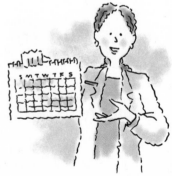

Spend at least an hour per month reviewing information and it will stay fresh.

Knowing isn't always understanding

It's possible for information to be memorized without being understood. With *rote memorization*, the information can be used only in situations similar to the one in which it was learned. For instance, you may have memorized a concept in chemistry when you were in high school, but because you didn't really understand it, you may find it impossible to apply that learning in your college chemistry class. Understanding a concept, as opposed to just memorizing it, helps to solidify the concept in your long-term memory. You might explain the concept to someone else to bolster your memory even further.

Try to apply

Nursing is an application discipline. Being able to merely recall a memorized fact doesn't mean you'll be able to apply it on a test or in the clinical setting. Think about how a particular fact or group of facts would be used in a client situation. What would the nurse do first? How would the care change if one aspect of the situation were to change? Use critical thinking exercises in your textbook or online to promote your ability to apply the content you've learned.

Using the depth gauge

The more deeply a topic is processed by the brain, the more solid is the long-term memory of that topic. Processing depth depends on how the learner processes the information and on a number of other factors, including the learner's:
• background knowledge
• desire for learning
• intended use of the information
• intensity of concentration
• level of interest in the topic
• overall attitude.

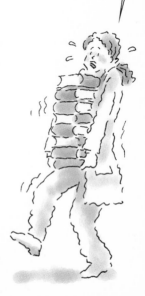

I have all sorts of study strategies at my disposal. It's just that I could use help carrying them.

Study strategies

By using a number of study strategies, you can give yourself the greatest chance to recall information later — on tests or in the clinical setting. Using different study strategies gives the brain more pathways to use when recalling information.
    Key study strategies include:
• using practice and repetition
• using spaced study
• minimizing interference and distractions
• associating familiar items with items to be remembered
• making lists
• using imagery.

Practice

In learning, practice makes permanent. Practice aids the storage of information in long-term memory. It also makes retrieval of information from long-term memory into working memory more automatic.

Rehearsal forms

Practice methods assume many forms, depending on the amount of time spent practicing, the depth of learning that takes place as a result, and the manner in which the information is learned. Rehearsal can take three forms:

 Auditory — repeating information aloud or in discussion

 Visual — reading information silently over and over

Semantic — writing or diagramming information repeatedly. Pay particular attention to the concept maps and diagrams in this book and in your textbooks, as well as those given to you by your instructors. They present information in a different format, allowing you to see relationships among concepts. Drawing concept maps yourself reinforces understanding.

Can you hear me now?

In general, auditory and semantic practices yield better results because they involve active processes rather than the more passive practice of silent reading. Rewriting information while saying it aloud can double your efficiency in learning. Learning takes place more readily as a result of active practices than passive ones.

Spaced study

Spaced study consists of alternating short study sessions with breaks. This method is also known as *distributed practice*. Study goals are set by time (for example, reading for at least 15 minutes) or task (for example, reading a minimum of three pages). After reaching these goals, the student takes a 5- to 15-minute break.

The secret to spaced study success

Spaced study works because:
- it rewards hard work
- work is completed in manageable portions
- work is completed under a deadline of time or task, so the time spent studying is spent efficiently
- working memory has limited capacity, so breaks provide time for information to be absorbed into long-term memory

- study breaks keep the student from confusing similar details when studying complex, interrelated information
- separate study sessions are more likely to involve different content cues. The greater the number of study sessions, the greater the likelihood that the content cues overlap with material on the test, thus improving recall.

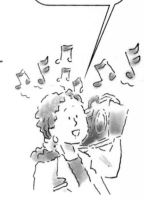

There's no static on this radio!

Interference reduction

Like radio signals creating static, *interference* occurs when new information conflicts with background knowledge. When two radio signals fall close to each other on the radiowave spectrum, it can be difficult to tune in one fully because of interference from the other. A similar kind of interference occurs in long-term memory. If you have many similar experiences or memories, you may find it difficult to retrieve information about a certain experience.

For instance, if you're trying to learn a large number of new terms and two of the terms are similar, you might have difficulty remembering either or both. To avoid interference, try to relate new information to previously learned information. Think about what makes the new information different from the previously learned information.

Take a breather

If you need to study the subjects one right after the other, take a break between the study sessions. When you return to study the second subject, try studying in a different place. Making different associations for each subject will help you and your brain organize information more efficiently.

Associations

To develop the necessary links among information and increase your ability to apply what you've learned, consider how to associate and organize information. (See *Developing associations*, page 30.) Applying knowledge to different situations is a critical aspect of learning that requires a deep understanding of the material. *Associations* form links between familiar items and items to be remembered. When established, the links become automatic.

Recalling a familiar item cues the recall of the other item. To be effective, associations must be personal, perhaps associating a song or smell with the item to be remembered.

Word games

Acronyms and acrostics each associate key information to an easily remembered word or phrase, thereby improving memory of the information.

Exercise your mind

Developing associations

Associating information you want to learn with information you already know can help you remember key pieces of information more easily. Use these questions to help you develop associations among study items.

- What, if anything, does the item remind you of?
- Does the item sound like a familiar word or rhyme with one?
- Can you link the item with a memory of a familiar location?
- Can you draw a picture to link your memory with the item?
- When you think of the item, can you visualize something familiar?
- Can you rearrange letters in the name to form an acronym?
- Can you form connections that make sense between one concept and another?

Pump up your long-term memory with acronyms!

Forming acronyms or acrostics can help in recalling lists of information. *Acronyms* are created from the first letter or the first few letters of each item on a list. *Roy G. Biv* is a commonly used acronym that stands for the colors of the rainbow in order (red, orange, yellow, green, blue, indigo, and violet). *HOMES* is another common acronym, this time for the names of the Great Lakes (Huron, Ontario, Michigan, Erie, and Superior). Acronyms need not be real words.

Acrostics are phrases or sentences represented on the vertical axis and are created from the first letter or first few letters of items on a list. For example, an acrostic representing the lines on the treble clef of a sheet of music is *Every Good Boy Does Fine*, which stands for the notes as they appear vertically, from the bottom up, on a treble clef: E-G-B-D-F.

In health care, one of the most famous acrostics is this one (or a variation of it) about the 12 cranial nerves: *On Old Olympus's Towering Tops, A Finn and a Swedish Girl Viewed Some Hops*, which stands for the olfactory, optic, oculomotor, trochlear, trigeminal, abducens, facial, sensorimotor (vestibulocochlear), glossopharyngeal, vagal, spinal accessory, and hypoglossal nerves.

Elaborate, please

Understanding how concepts can be connected with one another helps you learn by allowing for the elaboration of ideas. *Elaboration* enables you to reframe information in terms of what you already know about the topic. You provide your own logic from your knowledge of how the new information fits with previously learned information.

Lists

Lists serve as another memory aid. The arrangement of a list depends on your goals and the course emphasis and content. Sometimes an instructor suggests organizational structures for lists by identifying types of information to remember — for example, dates, names, and places.

Lists help organize ideas by categorizing information according to some commonality. Recalling the name of the organizing concept helps you remember the details located within it. The organization of information in the list depends on having a classification system of some kind. Because items relate to one another within the system, you can rearrange and reorganize information as needed to aid recall.

Imagery

People commonly think in images rather than in words. The use of visual aids in studying can help you recall familiar and unfamiliar information. In addition, images are stored differently in the brain than are words. Imagery provides an additional way to encode information. The brain stores four kinds of memories easily:

 patterns

 pictures

 rhymes

 stories.

Link 'em up

Mental associations link concrete objects with images (for example, a picture of a tree with the word *tree*) or abstract concepts with symbols (for example, a picture of a heart with the word *love*). Mental imagery also can be used to link unrelated objects, concepts, and ideas through visualization. For example, to remember which bone in the forearm is the radius, visualize yourself taking a patient's radial pulse. Then think to yourself that the end of the radius is located beneath the radial pulse.

Add a little color

You can use visual representations to help compress and synthesize class notes. Because visual representations of ideas are

Exercise your mind

Recall mapping

Recall mapping is a study technique that uses pictures to enhance memory. For example, you might need to remember a number of health care terms and their definitions. Here's how to perform recall mapping for a series of terms:

• Identify general headings under which the terms might fall.

• List appropriate terms under each heading.

• Draw two lines under each term. On the first line, draw a picture of an object that you can associate with the term or its meaning. On the second line, write the meaning of the term in your own words.

Studying the map

To study the terms using your recall map, cover the information below the term with a sheet of paper, and then try to remember the term's meaning. If you can't remember the meaning, slide the paper away to reveal the picture.

Seeing the drawing should prompt your recall of the meaning. If it doesn't, uncover the definition. Lastly, study the term again, recalling why you drew that particular picture. These illustrations show an example of a word map.

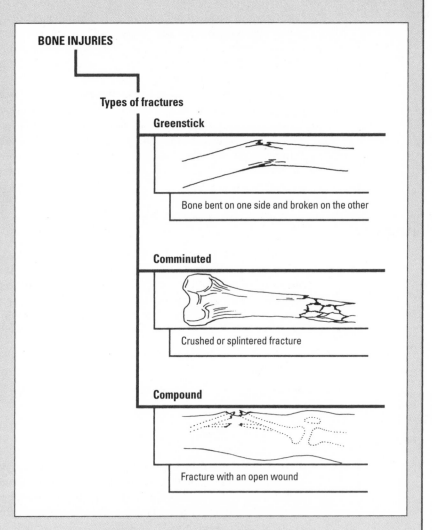

BONE INJURIES

Types of fractures

Greenstick

Bone bent on one side and broken on the other

Comminuted

Crushed or splintered fracture

Compound

Fracture with an open wound

processed by a different area of the brain than are words, they provide another way to recall information.

Adding meaningful doodles, colors, or symbols to your notes allows you to organize and then visualize information to be learned. A technique called *recall mapping* can be highly useful in this regard. (See *Recall mapping.*) When you use visual representations efficiently, you'll remember more information with less effort.

Improving memory skills

You can improve your memory skills through memory-boosting strategies, including:
- writing new information correctly
- using repetition
- using environmental cues
- understanding the information
- developing your own memorization techniques
- using vivid imagery
- having faith in yourself.

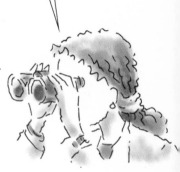

Paying attention to your surroundings can give your memory skills a big boost.

Look alive!

Being aware of everything around you is the first step in developing better recall. Be observant. Look for landmarks. Practice paying attention to the big things, and you'll become more attentive to the little ones too.

To remember information, the information must first be registered in your brain correctly. If a piece of information doesn't register, try to expose yourself to the information again. For example, if a new acquaintance's name doesn't register the first time you hear it, ask for the name again. Then repeat it to confirm it.

Now that makes sense!

Make sure you thoroughly understand what you want to remember. Information that makes sense to you and that you fully understand is easier to recall later. To boost your understanding of a topic, use several styles of learning. For instance, don't just read about the radius and ulna. Instead, read about them, watch a video about anatomy, draw a picture of the bones, manipulate your own arm, and talk about the location of the bones with peers. Using various methods of learning can enhance understanding and meaning and, as a result, improve recall.

Keep your eyes on the prize

To intensify your desire to recall information, keep a positive attitude about memory and recall. Believing that you can do something is an important step in actually doing it.

In addition, the more you keep your eyes on your overall goals, the more you can remember. The goal can serve as your incentive to remember information. The stronger the incentive, the stronger the mental connection and the longer lasting the memory.

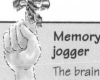

Memory jogger

The brain easily stores patterns, pictures, rhymes, and stories. Remember these categories easily by remembering:

Patty picked a rhyming story

to remember thoughts in all their glory.

The stranger, the better!

To make images in your mind easier to recall, make them more vivid. Think of the colors as being intensely bright. Make the image bigger. Associate a strong emotion to the picture. The more unusual or absurd the mental picture, the more likely that you'll be able to recall the information associated with it.

Here are other ideas for creating vivid images:

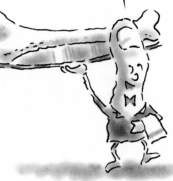

Picture this and you'll never forget that the radius is on my side (the thumb's side) of the forearm!

• Imagine some kind of action taking place, such as the taking of a pulse.
• Form an image of an object out of proportion to the object's actual size. Make the radius the size of a minivan!
• Exaggerate the object the way a caricature exaggerates the features of its subject.
• Substitute or reverse a normal role. For example, to remember that the radius is located on the thumb side of the forearm, imagine a huge thumb carrying the radius on a dinner tray at a restaurant.
• Practice word associations using mental pictures to remember items in a list. If you need to remember the names of middle ear bones — malleus (also called the *hammer*), incus (*anvil*), and stapes (*stirrup*)— imagine a cartoonish hammer duking it out with an anvil in a match refereed by a whistle-blowing stirrup. These word associations are memorable because they paint a bizarre picture.

Keep it simple

Probably the simplest method of remembering a piece of information is to associate the information with something familiar. You can recall one item because another item acts as a reminder. If, for example, you wanted to remember to take your anatomy and physiology textbook home to do an assignment, you might place a red sticky note on your assignment book.

Repetition...repetition...repetition...

Repetition is one of the most effective recall strategies of all. Repetition strengthens neural pathways and, with enough use, can create nearly indelible pathways. Don't depend on repetition alone, however. Use several strategies to make sure the memory remains intact.

Variety is the spice of life

Develop your own favorite memorization techniques, depending on the type of information that needs to be memorized. If you develop a unique memorization technique that works for you, then by all means continue to use it.

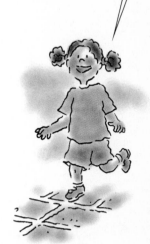

Feel like a kid again! Take a break, and play one of my favorite games!

As with all techniques, though, remember that you shouldn't rely on a single technique to learn new information, no matter how well that technique has served you in the past. Using a variety of techniques will serve you best in the long run.

Remember that expanding your arsenal of memorization techniques makes you a more flexible learner, which will allow you to learn a greater variety of material with less stress and wasted time.

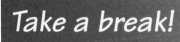

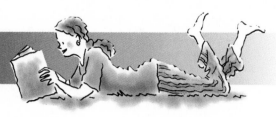

What's different?

Memory games were some of the first tools you used as a child to test your brain. List the ten differences between these two graphics, and check out your score on the next page!

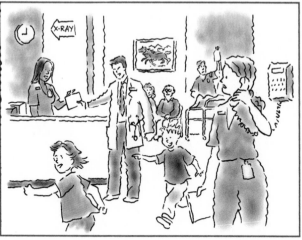

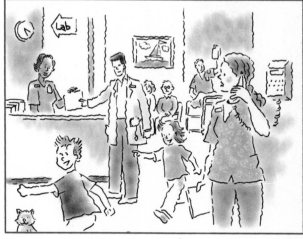

1. _____

2. _____

3. _____

4. _____

5. _____

6. _____

7. _____

8. _____

9. _____

10. _____

Answer key

1. The phone is a banana.
2. The little boy is now a little girl.
3. The little girl is now a little boy
4. The artwork on the wall is different.
5. The doctor's tie is missing.
6. The nurse's scrubs are different.
7. The time on the clock is different.
8. There's a cat in the emergency department.
9. The desk nurse's hair is a different length.
10. The "X-ray" on the sign now reads "Lab."

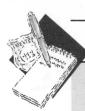

3

Managing your time

Just the facts

In this chapter, you'll learn:

♦ how a well-organized schedule is used to maximize studying efficiency

♦ how to set priorities effectively

♦ how to avoid burnout

♦ how procrastination can be overcome by effective planning and a positive approach to projects

♦ studying strategies and programs that improve learning skills.

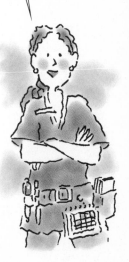

The right tools make short- and long-range planning a lot easier!

Schedules

The work habits of people who have achieved outstanding success invariably include a well-designed schedule. When facing several obligations at the same time, it becomes difficult to meet any of them. The purpose of scheduling isn't to feel constricted but, rather, to allow you to look ahead and free yourself from scholastic inefficiency and the anxiety that arises from not being prepared. Developing a course schedule can go a long way toward fulfilling those time management goals.

The "getting started" toolbox

The most successful scheduling technique for most students involves short-range and long-range planning. Develop a general schedule for each term, a specific but flexible schedule for each week, and a daily to-do list. The tools you'll need to get started include:

• a long-term (semester) calendar that can be posted where you study or carried with you to class and home or dorm

• a "week-at-a-glance" calendar that includes the current semester

- colorful pens or pencils for color-coding dates and tasks
- a notepad or stack of $3'' \times 5''$ lined cards or sticky notes for daily to-do lists.

Alternatively, you can use an all-in-one organizer system, such as a Day Timer or Day Runner. These systems generally include short-term and long-term calendars and daily to-do lists that can be replaced as needed.

Whichever format you choose, spend time at the beginning of the term planning and writing tests and assignments on the calendar. Review at least weekly, making adjustments as necessary.

Organizing a class schedule

The way you organize your class schedule affects the success you achieve during the term. If you organize your class schedule well, you can manage your time more effectively. To organize your class schedule properly, spread out class periods throughout the week, schedule difficult classes when you're most alert, strive for a balance between difficult and less-difficult courses each semester, and maintain flexibility throughout the schedule.

Spread the classes around

Some classes are scheduled on alternating days — Monday, Wednesday, and Friday, for instance. Some students may schedule all of their courses on those days, thinking that concentrating their class time and having a day or two free to study makes sense for time management. This arrangement, however, often results in being overworked and burned out on class days and then spending free days recuperating rather than studying. If possible, space your classes throughout the week.

Keep in mind that an efficient schedule fills the day as well as the week. Having sufficient time between classes gives you the opportunity to review information as soon as possible after class, which, in turn, gives you time to think through a lecture while the information is still fresh in your mind.

At many schools, nursing students don't have the ability to choose days and times for classes. If you find yourself unable to choose your class schedule, focus on adapting to the schedule you're given. Give yourself time to study and review information within the contraints of your schedule, and always check with faculty if you have a major conflict.

Tackling the tough classes

Your most difficult courses should be scheduled during the times you're most alert. If you prefer getting up early, schedule your most difficult course for the morning. If you do your best work after lunch, schedule your most difficult classes at that time.

If you have the option of scheduling a class on successive versus alternating days, consider the level of difficulty of the class and how interested you are in it. Difficulty level and interest in a topic affect the length of time you can concentrate on it. The more interested you are or the easier the content is for you, the longer you can sustain concentration on the topic.

> Try to balance your schedule. Balance the difficult courses with the easier ones.

Magical mix of courses

Although some courses must be taken in sequence, most curricula are somewhat flexible. Generally, course outlines are suggestions about how to spread mandatory and elective courses over one or more terms. Taking too many difficult courses at once can be overwhelming. Taking too many uninteresting classes can lead to boredom.

To offset either situation, balance courses that you look forward to attending with those you're less interested in, and balance difficult courses with easier courses.

Oh, those commitments

If you're like most students, you have personal commitments (such as holding a full-time or part-time job) or seasonal commitments (such as being a track athlete who trains in the spring). You may also have a hobby that dictates how much time you can devote to course work. Consider these activities and commitments when planning course work, and adjust your course schedule accordingly.

> Make time for hobbies *and* course work!

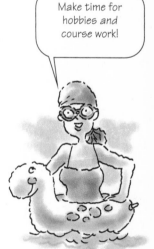

Check 'em out

You may have the option of taking a course with two or more different instructors. If the dates and times of each course fit your schedule, you'll need to decide with which instructor you'd like to take the class. If you don't know the instructors involved, check with other students who may have insight into those instructors, or with student government associations, which commonly monitor faculty performance and make results available to students.

Day-to-day time management

After determining your class schedule for the term, you need to turn your attention to managing your time each day. Start by setting up a calendar to record goals and major events. The purpose of such a calendar is to obtain an overview of long-term goals and commitments, which can help in planning short-term and daily activities.

Managing your calendar

Your calendar should include recreational as well as serious commitments. Using a calendar for the current year, mark off the months and days for the term in which you're currently enrolled. Put the calendar close to where you study so you can focus on your long-term objectives.

Use a calendar to record:
- midterm and final examination dates
- due dates for papers and other projects
- deadlines for completing each phase of lengthy projects
- test dates
- important extracurricular and recreational events
- deadlines for dropping and adding courses
- holidays, school vacations, and social commitments.

From start to finish

The beginning and end of each term are critical times for students.

Large amounts of content and course organizational material are commonly presented during the first few weeks of the term. Keep up with your readings and other work in this early period to set the pace for the term. If you start to fall behind or don't understand the content, talk with your instructor and your school's student support services. With their help in planning, you can stay on track.

The end of the term is also critical because students run out of time to bring their grades back up if they've fallen behind. Use your calendar to help spot possible distractions during these critical periods. Then plan how to eliminate the distractions or at least reduce their effects.

Is it hot in here?

Burnout results when a student works steadily without taking a sufficient number of breaks. The causes of burnout include fatigue, boredom, and stress.

Maintaining a balance between breaks and work time — and planning for both — helps avoid burnout. A break doesn't have to be recreational; it can be a change from one task to another. For example, switching from an anatomy assignment to a reading

Taking a relaxing break is one way to cool down a bad case of burnout!

assignment in your fundamentals textbook can relieve boredom and, thus, prevent burnout. Such planning also decreases interruptions during prime study time.

Another way to avoid burnout is to retain flexibility in your daily schedule. If you schedule commitments too tightly during the day, you won't have time to complete your goals and, as a result, may feel defeated for failing to do what you had planned.

Setting priorities

Setting priorities is a critical task for every student. You'll need to set priorities appropriately in school and in the clinical setting as well. You'll need to set priorities for tasks, class attendance, and homework.

Tasks

A student with several tasks that have the same deadline may switch back and forth from one task to another, giving the illusion of progress. Changing tasks too often, however, wastes time because you lose momentum. For a time after the transition from one project to another, you may still be thinking about the old project when you should be concentrating on the new one. Furthermore, after returning to the first task, you have to review the material where you left off and remember what steps remained before the task could be finished.

So many tasks, so little time

You can avoid this problem by determining how much time you have available in any one period. If you have an hour or less, work on only one task; only alternate tasks if you have more than an hour. Even then, most of your attention should be focused on completing a single task (or a large portion of it), which can provide a sense of satisfaction and move you steadily toward completion of your goals.

It's rude to interrupt!

If you interrupt work on a long-term project to work on another task, write a few notes about the long-term project before moving to the new task. Write down the goal of the task and a list of questions to be answered or objectives to be completed. You might jot down what steps you plan to perform next so that, when you return to the task, you can pick up where you left off right away. Also, be sure to store all materials related to the first task in the same place so you don't have to search for them when you return to the task.

Attending class

During class, the instructor highlights the most important concepts, elaborates on information found in assigned readings, and shapes the student's understanding of the material. Instructors focus on application, analysis, and synthesis of ideas in their lectures and classroom work. Instructors use class time to present the material they think is most important for understanding the course.

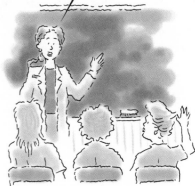

I already covered that at the beginning of class.

To get the most out of class time, arrive on time and don't leave early. Instructors commonly use the first 5 minutes of class to make important announcements, and the last 5 minutes to summarize material or explain assignments.

Bring other assignments or readings to class in case the instructor is late or you have an unexpected break. Know the policies of your school and instructor regarding class attendance and lateness. Because professional behavior is expected of nursing students, there may be special requirements or consequences related to that behavior or the lack of it.

Risky business

Missing a class is risky. Each time you miss a class, you face the possibility that questions on the next test will relate to material covered in the class you missed.

Many students assume they can safely miss a class here and there because they pay close attention to their reading assignment. The problem with that approach is that many instructors don't use only the reading material to construct lecture notes and create classroom activities and discussions.

Instructors commonly base classroom material on their own experiences and on sources not readily available to the student, such as journal articles, educational newsletters, and other non-textbook sources of information. Even if an instructor bases her classroom activities entirely on textbook readings, you would still miss explanations of new ideas and the further development of existing content.

The body-brain split

Here's another reason not to skip class: Learning continues outside the classroom. After class, you continue to think about the material. You may be walking home from class, showering, or doing the laundry when you come up with a question to ask or clarify in your mind a statement made in class. Just because your body is no longer located in a classroom doesn't mean your brain has finished analyzing material covered in that classroom. Give your mind a chance to help you learn; attend every class.

The bitter end

The worst time to miss a class is at the end of the semester. Some instructors use the last few classes of the semester to review and outline the entire course or to discuss information to be covered on the final examination. Some instructors even go so far as to tell — or at least hint at — exactly what material the students should study for the final examination.

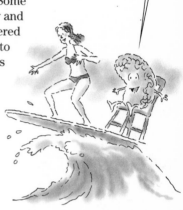

Just because she's out there having fun doesn't mean that I'm done working!

Even so, some students feel overwhelmed with studying for final examinations and end up trading class time for study time. If you schedule your study time well, you can avoid feeling the need to skip class to study. If you're truly unable to attend a class, however, ask another student if you can borrow her notes and get copies of classroom handouts for that day. That way, you'll at least be exposed to some of the material covered in class.

Doing homework

Homework assignments typically fall into two categories: written and reading assignments. Written assignments provide an instructor with immediate feedback about how much work the student has done and how well she has understood it.

Although reading assignments don't provide immediate feedback, instructors generally consider them as important as written assignments for understanding a particular subject. Many instructors include questions on reading assignments on quizzes and tests, or ask questions in class based on assigned readings. The responses of the students help the instructor gauge the effectiveness of the assignments and whether the students have actually read the material.

Eh, what's next, Doc?

To gain the most value from homework assignments, you first need to find out what the assignments are for the course. Most instructors distribute a syllabus or an outline at the start of each course. These documents explain content to be covered in the course and what expectations the instructor has for the student. Some instructors also distribute reading and written homework assignments for each course. If you don't receive such an outline, approach your instructor and ask what material you should read for the next few classes. Then create your own outline, and put the assignments into your organizer so you can plan your daily and weekly schedule properly.

My dog ate my homework!

Family and other responsibilities sometimes take precedence over schoolwork. In those situations, try to balance your schedule by not overdoing it in one area at the expense of another. Postponing certain homework assignments for a short time may free up enough time to fulfill family obligations or other responsibilities. Having the support of your employer, fellow workers, and family can prove critical in this regard. However, avoid postponing homework routinely. Doing so can put you so far behind in your studies that you won't be able to catch up.

Handling procrastination

Everyone procrastinates, some more so than others. In the end, procrastination results in wasted time, missed opportunities, poor performance, self-deprecation, and increased stress. Procrastinators often spend more time worrying than working.

Excuses, excuses!

People who procrastinate place low-priority tasks ahead of high-priority ones and then offer excuses for not doing the high-priority task, including:

- I'll wait until I'm in the mood.
- I feel like celebrating because I finished reading one chapter.
- I'll think about it tomorrow.
- There's plenty of time to get it done.
- I don't know where to begin.
- I work best under pressure.
- I have too many other things to do first.

Students may procrastinate to avoid tasks that seem boring or difficult, or they may put off working on a task because they doubt their ability to do the task in the first place. In addition, a student may wait until all available resources have been reviewed before completing a task. Regardless of the cause, procrastination needs to be identified and then overcome to succeed as a student. (See *Breaking the procrastination habit.*)

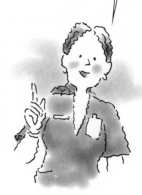

Here's the low-down on low-priority tasks. Don't put them ahead of high-priority ones.

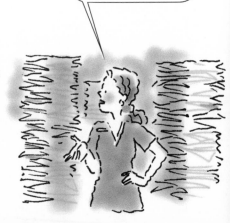

I've broken 18 large tasks into about a gazillion smaller parts. Gee, I feel much better!

Advice from the experts

Breaking the procrastination habit

Procrastination habits can be hard to break but not impossible. Here are some tips for breaking your procrastination habits.

Motivators

• On one side of a sheet of paper, write your reasons for not doing something. On the other side, challenge the excuse with logic. For example, if your reason for not starting your Dosage Calculations project is that you aren't in the mood, you might counter with, "Well, you may *never* be in the mood and the job will *never* get done unless you do it."

• Make up a list of self-motivating statements, such as "It's now or never," "No time like the present," or "Never put off until tomorrow what you can do today." Then repeat them whenever you feel like postponing a task.

• Recognize that the negative predictions you may make about a project aren't facts. Focus on the positive steps you can take toward reaching your goals, no matter how difficult those goals might be.

• Commit to complete each task. Promise yourself, a friend, or a relative that you'll get the task done. A promise to a third person can serve as a powerful motivator.

Goals and priorities

• Design clear goals, and then establish a realistic timetable to complete each one.

• Set priorities. Write down all the things that need to be done for a project in order of their importance. The greater the importance, the higher the priority.

• Break down large, complex projects into smaller, more manageable parts. For example, make an outline for a written report before composing it.

• Use your weekly schedule and daily to-do lists to keep yourself organized. Check off tasks after completion.

• Pinpoint where your delays typically start, and then focus on overcoming procrastination during those critical times.

• Write reminders to yourself about projects to be completed, and display them in conspicuous places.

Rewards

• Reward yourself. Self-reinforcement can have a powerful effect on developing a "do it now" attitude.

• Promise yourself to give up something important if you fail to meet your goal and to go someplace special if you *do* meet your goal.

Give it a try

When you recognize that you're procrastinating, try doing what you're thinking about postponing for just a few minutes. After you've started the task, you're likely to continue working on it.

Parcel it out

When you face several deadlines in the same week, it can be difficult to prioritize and get started on a task. In these cases, parcel the work, setting apart small tasks that can be accomplished quickly. Completing several small tasks provides positive reinforcement and moves you closer and closer to your goal.

Get real!

Some students fail to start projects because they set impossibly high standards for themselves and are afraid they won't live up to their own expectations. Other students refuse to finish a project until they believe it's perfect, a goal they may never reach. In either case, you should weigh the consequences of handing in what you believe is a flawed project with the consequences of not handing in a project at all. Understand that a passing grade for an imperfect assignment beats a zero for not handing in an assignment at all. Use this knowledge as an impetus for getting the project completed at all costs.

Down with distractions!

If a student procrastinates because she can't concentrate enough to get started on a project, she needs to remove the distractions from her study area or move to an area with fewer distractions. When undertaking a project, make sure that reference materials are nearby so that you don't interrupt your work flow to find a particular resource.

To study or not to study?

Sometimes uncertainty can cause apathy and indecisiveness and, consequently, procrastination. For instance, if you aren't sure which topic you should choose for a project, you'll have a harder time making a commitment to the project and an easier time putting off getting started. To avoid procrastination caused by uncertainty, keep in mind that decisiveness is a trait of an effective leader and a successful student. Brainstorming for ideas with other students, asking your instructor for suggestions on a topic, or researching several topics that may interest you can help you decide on a topic and move you toward fulfilling your goals.

Review your goals

Lack of clear, specific goals is often a subtle cause of procrastination. If you're unsure of your goals, you'll have little reason to begin or complete a project. Likewise, if you become very involved in working on one assignment, you may forget due dates for other commitments. Establishing long-term and short-term goals — and then periodically reviewing them — can help provide direction to the tasks you perform and keep you on track during unusually busy periods.

Preparing to study

Effective studying doesn't just happen. It involves carefully select-ing a study site, maintaining proper lighting, settling into a com-fortable position, and putting yourself into the right frame of mind.

Selecting a study area

To find the right study area, look for a distraction-free spot where you can arrange your study materials properly. Make sure it has adequate lighting, is set at the right temperature, and is located among pleasant surroundings.

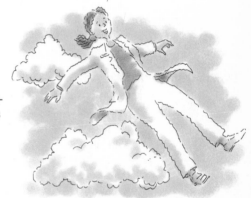

A good study area is calm, comfortable, and free from distractions. There is, however, such a thing as *too comfortable!*

Distraction-free site

Before you begin to study, find a calm, comfort-able place to study. As you select your study site, choose an area with the fewest distractions. (See *Distraction-free study areas.*) After you find a study site you enjoy using, keep using it for subse-quent study sessions. Using the same area creates familiarity and helps you begin studying as soon as you settle into the area.

Exercise your mind

Distraction-free study areas

Select two or three areas you think may be suitable to use as study areas. Then choose the area that gets the most favorable responses to these questions:
• Will I be interrupted by other people?
• Are there too many reminders of things that don't have anything to do with studying?
• Is a loud radio or television being played here?
• Does the telephone ring too often?
• Can I be here at regular intervals?
• Is the temperature comfortable or, if not, can I control the temperature?
• Can I smell cooking odors here?

Study arrangement

Next, find the arrangement for studying you most enjoy. For most students, a desk with a comfortable, straight-backed chair makes the ideal study arrangement. You can arrange your study materials on the desk and easily reach them whenever necessary. Other students feel most comfortable in a large chair or sofa, with their books and other study materials spread out on the floor at their feet.

Don't get too relaxed

You could sit cross-legged in the middle of your bed with your study materials all around, but it's probably not a good idea. You're already familiar with your bed as a sleeping place, and you may get sleepy. Sitting under a tree with a gentle breeze blowing in a quiet place seems like a good idea, but not when the gentle breeze becomes a distraction, ruffling papers and making you constantly lose your place in your notes. Choose your study arrangement carefully, weighing the value of the comfort it provides with its ability to meet your study needs.

It's habit forming

To help you decide which study arrangement and study area are right for you, ask yourself these questions:
- Do I have sufficient work space?
- Can I keep the work space uncluttered?
- Do I have adequate lighting?
- Am I in a position that supports my back and eliminates muscle strain?
- Are there as few distractions as possible in the area?

Whichever study arrangement you choose, stay with it. Get into the habit of assuming your study position so you can get down to the business of studying quickly, with few distractions.

Lighting

Use either natural or incandescent lighting for your study area, not fluorescent lighting. Your eyes are less likely to tire under direct light, such as that from an incandescent lamp, than under indirect light.

Direct lighting is best, keeping eye fatigue at its lowest. Keep the light from shining in your eyes by using overhead light or lighting from behind. The light should shine evenly on your work.

> **Memory jogger**
> When you're trying to find a place to study, a;ways remember to check out the **SALT** beforehand:
> **S**urroundings
> **A**rrangement
> **L**ighting
> **T**emperature.

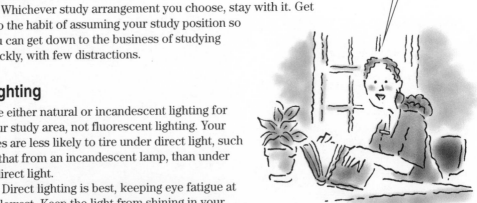

> For studying, nothing beats natural light.

Temperature

Choose a study area that isn't too warm. Heat stress can decrease accuracy, speed, dexterity, and physical acuity. For most efficient studying, keep your study area cool — between 65° and 70° F (18° and 21° C).

Surroundings

Pleasant surroundings can greatly enhance study effectiveness. The sensations experienced while studying can be used later to trigger associations at test time. Pleasant surroundings also stimulate alertness. When creating the environment of your study site, focus on surrounding yourself with pleasant music, stimulating odors, and oxygen-providing plants.

Ahh, the pleasing sounds of Mozart...

Minimize noise distractions while you study so you won't be disturbed. Screen your telephone calls with an answering machine. Leave the television off. You may also consider adding white noise to your environment. Instrumental music, the sound of a bubbling aquarium, and muted street sounds are examples of white noise. White noise helps cover distracting background sounds, such as the sounds of traffic or your roommate talking on the phone, and fills in periods of silence. In silence, even the sound of your own tapping pencil can be annoying.

Among the forms of white noise you can use, soothing background music is preferred. Low levels of background music can promote relaxed alertness, which stimulates learning. In addition, music induces an emotional response that can be associated with a memory and improve later recall.

...And the scent of peppermint

The two scents that most positively stimulate attention and memory are lemon and peppermint. These scents can be found in oils, candles, room fresheners, and many other products. Other scents also exert an enhancing effect on mental alertness and relaxation. (See *Scents and the mind*, page 50.)

Gotta get some green (plants, that is)

Studying in an area where healthy plants are located can actually foster learning. Green plants remove pollutants from the air and can raise oxygen levels enough to increase productivity by as much as 10%.

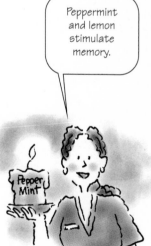

Peppermint and lemon stimulate memory.

Scents and the mind

Certain scents have been specifically identified as influencing mental alertness and relaxation. This chart lists those scents and the ways they can affect your studying.

Scent	Effect
basil	increased mental alertness
chamomile	enhanced relaxation
cinnamon	increased mental alertness
lavender	enhanced relaxation
lemon	increased mental alertness
orange	enhanced relaxation
peppermint	increased mental alertness
rose	enhanced relaxation

Physical comfort

Your physical comfort affects your attitude about studying. When studying, make sure you assume a comfortable posture, use an appropriate reading angle, and move around periodically to enhance study effectiveness.

Sit up, like your mom used to tell you

Read while sitting in an upright position with your back straight or bent slightly forward. Other postures — particularly lying down — impair alertness and concentration.

Get the right angle

To decrease eyestrain, hold reading material at about a 45-degree angle from the flat surface of your desk or table to give you a clear view of the whole page. Reading material should also be kept at least 15″ away from your eyes.

Get moving

Walking around periodically when studying can enhance the ability of the brain to learn new information and retain information. On average, standing increases blood flow to the brain by 5% to

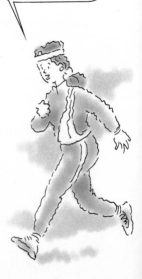

Walk around and stretch every now and then when studying. Your brain can use the oxygen.

15%. The greater the blood flow to the brain, the more oxygen it receives and the greater the stimulation of the neurons. So take a break about every hour to walk around, particularly if you need to ponder a point or repeat some facts to yourself. Do some stretching exercises as well to increase circulation and decrease muscle fatigue in the shoulders.

Getting started

One of the biggest challenges to effective studying is getting started. The first step in meeting that challenge is to break down large tasks into smaller ones. Several small tasks seem more achievable than one overwhelming one, and each smaller accomplishment provides moral support to finish the other tasks.

Set the compass

By taking small steps in the direction you want to go, you may end up at your destination sooner than you thought. For instance, you may not feel like reading your assignment, but if you tell yourself that you'll read for 5 minutes, at least you'll get a little reading done. After a few minutes, tell yourself that you'll read for a few more minutes, and so on. Pretty soon, you'll have read for half an hour or maybe even an hour and be well on your way to accomplishing — if not finishing — your assignment.

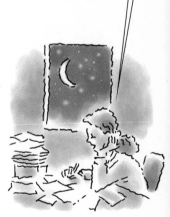

Ask yourself, "Why am I studying this? What's my goal? When can I go to bed?"

Plot the course

When beginning a study session, set a course for your studying or establish a purpose for it. Ask yourself, "What do I want to get out of this session? What do I need to know from the material?" After skimming the material, decide how deeply you need to become involved with it. You may be responsible for detailed knowledge and intricate notes or you may need only a passing acquaintance with the material. Either way, plot your course before you start.

Dump those dastardly distractions

Remove the usual distractions — the telephone, television, and talk radio. Take care of your personal distractions, such as being hungry or feeling hot. Schedule your study time so that it doesn't conflict with another activity you really want to do. Thinking about what you're missing can be a distraction in itself.

Find the right time to study, when you're feeling most efficient and receptive to information. Take a short break every hour to keep your study time energized. When concentration begins to lag, it's time for a break.

Special study programs

Since the 1940s, study programs have been popular tools for helping students improve their studying efficiency. Four of the currently popular programs are:

- SQ4R reading-study system
- PSQ5R method
- reciprocal teaching
- metalearning.

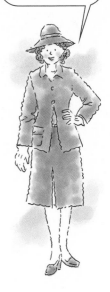

Since the 1940s, study tools have been helping students.

SQ4R reading-study system

The SQ4R reading-study system involves six steps:

Survey. Gather information necessary to formulate study goals.

Question. Formulate questions to be answered.

Read. Seek answers for the questions you raised.

Reflect. Think about what the text is trying to explain or teach you.

Recite. Ask your original questions and recite the answer to yourself. If you can't recite the answer, read the material again. Recitation can be particularly interactive when done with another person.

Review. Synthesize the reading material's meaning as a whole by determining whether you answered all your original questions and met all the goals you set forth after previewing the material. Another way to review involves answering questions posed by the author at the beginning or end of the material.

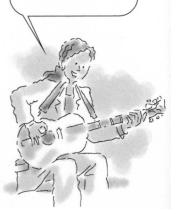

Survey, question, read, reflect, recite, review. I give it an 8. It's got a beat, but you can't dance to it.

PSQ5R method

The PSQ5R method, a system similar to the SQ4R system, involves eight steps:

Purpose. Determine your purpose for reading.

Survey. Preview the material quickly.

Question. Raise questions you think the reading should answer.

Read selectively. Read with your purpose and questions in mind.

Recite. Mentally repeat what you've learned as you go along.

Reduce-record. Write what you've learned in outline, or reduced, form.

Reflect. Mentally elaborate on what you've learned, comparing the material to previously learned material, categorizing it, or otherwise reorganizing the material.

Review. Survey your "reduced" notes (the outline) within 24 hours to enhance your knowledge of the material.

Reciprocal teaching

In *reciprocal teaching*, the student is taught to:
- summarize the content of a passage
- ask a question about the central point
- clarify the difficult parts of the material
- predict what will come next.

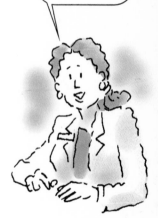

In reciprocal teaching, the student becomes the teacher.

Shhh...it's silent reading

Reciprocal teaching starts when you and the instructor silently read a short passage in a book or journal. Then the instructor provides a model by summarizing, questioning, clarifying, and predicting based on the reading. You'll then read another passage, but this time you'll assume the instructor's role by summarizing, questioning, clarifying, and predicting. The instructor may prompt you by giving clues, guidance, and encouragement to help you master these strategies.

Easy on the shift

To make reciprocal teaching effective, the shift from the instructor having control of the teaching process to you having the control must be gradual. Furthermore, the instructor must match the difficulty of the task to your own particular abilities.

Metalearning

Metalearning is a method of learning that involves asking yourself a series of questions:
- Why am I reading or listening to this?
- What's the overall content?
- What are the orientation questions?
- What's important here?
- Can I paraphrase or summarize the information?
- How can I organize the information?
- How can I draw the information?

- Can I associate the information?
- How does the information fit what I know?

Setting the stage

In the metalearning process, state your purpose briefly. Your purpose and goals set the stage for your study session. In the case of a lecture, ask yourself what you want to get out of the class. Try to anticipate what's coming next.

Sneak preview

Preview the material before reading or attending the lecture. For long or complicated material, translate your preview into a chapter map or outline. You may also want to write what you know about the topic and what you'd like to know or expect to learn about it. This type of warm-up starts the process of generating questions, makes you aware of what you don't know about a topic, puts you on the lookout for answers to questions, and provides a resource on which to draw later. After previewing the material, summarize the chapter in a few sentences and outline brief answers to whatever review questions may be included in the book.

Getting oriented

Be on the lookout for orientation questions, which commonly appear on tests. An *orientation question* provides background information about a topic or concept and can take many forms, including those that ask about definitions, examples, types, relationships, or comparisons.

The purpose for identifying orientation questions is to see how many questions you can ask about the material and how many different answers you can create for each. Don't be afraid to guess at the answer. Later, when you find out the actual answer, compare it with the one you gave. If you don't find the answer to your question, try looking in a different source.

To focus or skim — that is the question

Identify which information you should focus on, skim, or ignore. If you can't decide whether something is important, assume it is. Pay attention to your initial responses. If something surprises or confuses you, there may be a gap in your understanding of the information.

Each subject contains important terms you should know. Textbooks typically call your attention to them with italic or bold print or include the term in a glossary. Isolated facts or other details may be important — depending on your purpose for studying.

In other words...

Paraphrasing a concept — putting it into your own words — can help you better understand the concept and immediately identify

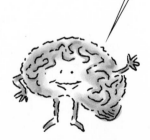

When you organize information, I can put it into groups or categories. Then you'll see the connections!

gaps in your learning. If you can't paraphrase a concept, you probably don't understand it well. To paraphrase effectively, use your own words and as few words as possible.

Making a connection

Organizing information allows your brain to place pieces of information into groups or categories so you can see patterns, connections, and relationships. Try to keep the number of groups manageable — fewer than 10 — so the information doesn't become too complicated to remember.

For example, if you need to learn the differences among several drugs, you might create categories that group the drugs by indications or adverse reactions only. That way, you can study the drugs in groups according to something they have in common, rather than studying them separately.

You might also consider organizing the information visually by using a mind-mapping technique. By writing the associations you're making among pieces of information, you're making a record of your natural thought processes about the information and will be more prepared to recall it later.

A picture is worth a thousand words

Representing information as pictures can be a great help in building understanding. Draw a picture of the information. The process of drawing the information can improve your understanding of the information and help move it into your long-term memory.

Associating new information with a song, rhyme, odor, or other environmental trigger can ease later recall. Use association and other memory-enhancing techniques to help retention and recall.

Your accumulated knowledge and understanding of the material help you decide what's important and condense new information into easier-to-manage pieces. If you already have a solid foundation of knowledge about the topic, you can more easily learn new aspects of the topic.

Engage the brain

Raising other questions can also help engage your brain and enhance retention and later recall. Some of these questions include:
• How is this information significant?
• What does it tell us about other things?
• Is this a fact or someone's opinion?
• How can this be verified?
• Does it depend on a particular point of view?
• What if…?
• Where have I seen something like this before?
• What does that suggest about this?
• What does this remind me of?

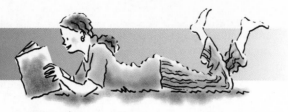

Take a break!

Timing is everything

Scheduling all your activities — as well as your studies — can be quite a task! See if you can help this student schedule her activities. Remember to schedule some time for meals and some downtime so she doesn't suffer burnout!

- Meet with study group to prepare for dosage calc test . . . . 2 hours
- Bake cookies for dosage calc study group . . . . ½ hour
- Chemistry class . . . . 9-10:30 a.m.
- Practice tennis for match . . . . 1 hour
- Proofread fundamentals paper and turn in . . . . 1 hour
- Take a bath and relax! . . . . as long as possible!
- Read 25 pages for med-surg nursing course . . . . 1 hour
- Do laundry! . . . . 1½ hours
- Watch part of roommate's lacrosse game . . . . 4-6 p.m.

Tomorrow

8 a.m.	4 p.m.
8:30 a.m.	4:30 p.m.
9 a.m.	5 p.m.
9:30 a.m.	5:30 p.m.
10 a.m.	6 p.m.
10:30 a.m.	6:30 p.m.
11 a.m.	7 p.m.
11:30 a.m.	7:30 p.m.
12 noon	8 p.m.
12:30 p.m.	8:30 p.m.
1 p.m.	9 p.m.
1:30 p.m.	9:30 p.m.
2 p.m.	10 p.m.
2:30 p.m.	10:30 p.m.
3 p.m.	11 p.m.
3:30 p.m.	11:30 p.m.

4

Textbook and classroom strategies

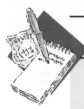

Just the facts

In this chapter, you'll learn:

♦ why effective reading skills are critical for success in studying, and how they can be improved with the consistent application of basic reading strategies

♦ how to prepare for a lecture ahead of time and why you should review your notes after lectures

♦ why using the principles of active reading and listening can improve comprehension.

Reading skills

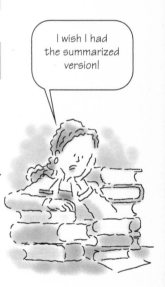

I wish I had the summarized version!

Students receive more than 75% of their course information from printed materials. This is why solid reading skills are essential for successful studying. Effective reading skills involve strategies to improve comprehension and reading speed.

Comprehension techniques

Reading and understanding course material provides support for lectures and classroom activities and leads to a thorough understanding of the topic under study. Improving reading comprehension involves skimming for ideas, using active reading skills, and summarizing the material.

Skimming for ideas

The first step in reading a chapter in a textbook is to look it over without trying to read every word. *Skimming* the chapter gives you an idea of the content and shows you how the material is organized. By thinking about the structure before actually reading the material, you use your brain to organize the learning to come, which improves your ability to understand the content and recall information in the chapter.

Getting to know you

Before reading a chapter in detail, look at the illustrations and read the captions. Then read the introductory paragraph and all the headings in the chapter. Lastly, read the chapter summary.

Use the same skimming techniques to read an entire book. First, look at the title page. Read about the author on the book jacket or on the *About the Author* page. Read the preface or other introductory material. Examine the table of contents to obtain a better idea of the book's content. Review the pages, noting emphasized words in bold or italics. Lastly, read vocabulary or glossary terms listed in the chapters or at the end of the book as appropriate.

A picture is worth a thousand words

Review all graphs, charts, tables, and illustrations. This supplemental content is intended to expand on or clarify the material covered in the main text, so use it to your advantage.

Experience breeds familiarity

Reading comprehension is enhanced when the reading material relates to your own background. For example, an experienced X-ray technician could most likely read faster and more readily understand a chapter about the advantages of using contrast medium in certain procedures. The technician's background gives her knowledge of relevant vocabulary and an ability to more quickly understand connections among concepts. As a result, she can more easily comprehend the material. (See *Improving your reading comprehension.*)

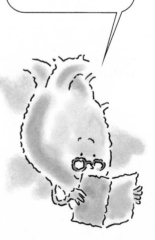

That cardiovascular system stuff was getting pretty complicated, so I decided to go back to the basics.

Back to the basics

To more easily understand material about a complex topic, try reading less advanced material on the same subject, listening to a lecture on it, or attending a seminar on a related topic.

There's a pattern here

Understanding how the text itself is organized can help you focus on the most important parts of the text. Common structural components include:

• subject development or *definition text structure*, which identifies a concept and lists its supporting details (These paragraphs are usually found at the beginning of major sections.)
• enumeration or *sequence text*, in which major points are listed by number or in sequence, and are commonly preceded by such clue words as *first, second, next,* and *then*

Advice from the experts

Improving your reading comprehension

Improving your reading comprehension doesn't have to be an impossible dream. Following these guidelines can help you more readily comprehend every reading assignment you have:

• Keep your purpose for reading squarely in mind.

• If the main idea is unstated, identify the topic by looking for repetitions of key words or phrases.

• Retrieve the background knowledge necessary to understand the text; use such strategies as looking up unknown words and referring to less advanced resources.

• Restate the main idea through paraphrasing, summarizing, or synthesizing.

• *compare-and-contrast text*, which expresses relationships between two or more ideas (Comparisons show how ideas are similar; contrasting statements show how they're different.)
• *cause-and-effect text*, which shows how one idea or event results from another idea or event.

Using active reading skills

Active reading fosters comprehension by involving more than one sense. To become a more active reader:
• read aloud
• take notes on the material you've read
• formulate some questions you'd like answered while you read
• think about the important points as outlined by the table of contents
• avoid arguing with the author when reading (you can analyze the text later)
• mark areas you'd like to read again.

While you're alert

Read during parts of the day when you feel comfortable, alert, and unhurried. If you know you have to read 25 pages today and that you get sleepy after lunch, avoid trying to complete your reading after lunch. Instead, choose a time when you're feeling more alert. Likewise, don't try to read too much at once. If you've been reading for a long time and begin to feel your concentration slipping, take a 5-minute break.

Distraction-free zone

Watching television, listening to music with lyrics, and engaging in numerous otherwise enjoyable activities can be distracting when trying to study. Avoid distractions by finding a quiet place to read. Sit at a desk or in a straight-backed chair bathed in natural or incandescent light. Try to avoid getting too comfortable and, as a result, becoming sleepy. Have a healthy snack and keep water handy to stave off hunger and thirst.

The handy highlighter

If you own the book you're reading, use a highlighter to mark important ideas. (See *Power-reading symbols.*) If you don't own the book, use colored sticky notes for marking key areas. In either case, don't overdo it. Marking up too much text makes the material meaningless after a while.

Keep these highlighting tips in mind:

• When buying a used text, never choose one that has already been highlighted or otherwise marked up by another student.

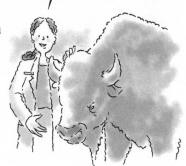

It's easy to get distracted by everyday ordinary things — television, music, a buffalo in your kitchen. Of course, I could always say a buffalo ate my homework!

Advice from the experts

Power-reading symbols

Using shortcuts for labeling text can help you read faster while still understanding the text. This table shows commonly used symbols for labeling text.

Symbol	Meaning
ex	example or experiment
form	formula
MI	main idea
! or *	important information
→	results in, leads to, steps in a sequence
(1), (2), (3)	important points
circled word	process summary
?	disagree or unclear
term	important term
summ	summary
{}	certain pieces of information relate
opin	author's opinion, rather than fact
∴	therefore

Advice from the experts

Marking and labeling text

Marking and labeling text can help you retain knowledge about the reading you've done and make later reference easier. Remember these points when marking and labeling text:

• Read a paragraph or section completely before marking anything.

• Mark points that answer questions you may have had before reading.

• Number lists, reasons, or other items that occur in a series or sequence.

• Identify important terms, dates, places, and names.

• Write main idea summaries, questions, and other comments in the margins.

• Put a question mark beside unclear or confusing information.

• Put a star or exclamation point beside information your instructor emphasizes in class, possible test questions, or what seems to be extremely important information.

• Write comments on the table of contents or make your own table of contents of important topics inside the front cover of the book or on the title page.

• If you skimmed the material before reading it, use your marks to note details that provide answers to your questions.

• Mark material you believe the instructor considers most important.

• Consider the difficulty of the language when deciding what content to mark. (See *Marking and labeling text.*) Subject depth, the number of details given, and overall vocabulary affect how much you understand.

Keep in mind that highlighters and sticky notes are *indexing tools;* they can help you find information, but they can't help you *learn* the information unless you do some follow-up work. Whenever you mark a section of your book, make sure you do something with it later, such as writing a summary of highlighted information or drawing a chart or diagram to summarize the information.

Zooming in

Every chapter has a central premise, and every paragraph within that chapter presents at least one main idea. The main ideas and supporting details of each paragraph support the central premise of the chapter.

In a typical paragraph, the *topic sentence* tells you the main idea. The topic sentence usually appears at the beginning or end of the paragraph but may appear anywhere. Pay particular attention to topic sentences, highlighting the sentence or parts of the sentence as appropriate.

So what you're saying is...

Take notes while you read. If you can rephrase the material, then you probably understand it. Comprehension builds on itself. Some concepts (in math, for example) must be understood before you can move on. One method of note "rephrasing" involves drawing graphics of the material. Graphics are sometimes more memorable than words, and the act of drawing them will give your memory an extra boost.

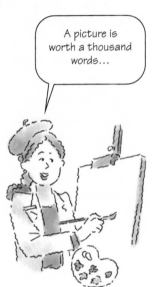

A picture is worth a thousand words...

Getting personal

The active reader assimilates information to relate to her own experience, thus making the information more easily remembered because it's more personal. The more personal the information, the more meaningful the material. Make the material more meaningful.

• Make associations of personal relevance. For example, perhaps an important date can be associated with a birth date.

• Allow it to evoke an emotional response. A deep emotional response to information or even something that strikes you as funny can make the information more interesting and, therefore, more entrenched in memory.

• Take advantage of your brain's ability to recall pictures, graphics, and illustrations. Draw out what you learn; make patterns, doodles, and drawings that make sense to *you*.

Criticism counts

Read critically, asking yourself questions about the text. Question the authority of the author or the reliability of the information provided. Questioning the content forces you to think critically about the information, which may open doors to greater understanding of the content and improve retention. Here are examples of critical questions:

• How can I apply this information to the care of a patient?
• How does this information relate to what I studied last week?
• Does the information validate ideas in other resources or contradict other reading?
• Under what circumstances were the data collected?
• How was the information verified?
• Do inconsistencies exist in the information?
• How does the author answer his own questions?
• Has the author made any assumptions?
• Are the author's statements based on knowledge, facts, experiences, or opinions?
• Is the author being objective?

- Do I disagree with the author? Why?
- If I were playing "devil's advocate," what questions would I ask the author? What examples would I include that the author hasn't?
- What do I want to know that the author hasn't told me?

Calling Mr. Webster...stat!

If you come across a word you've never seen, don't understand, or can't pronounce, look it up in a dictionary. However, first try to derive the meaning of the word from its context in the sentence and from its root words, prefixes, and suffixes. Try to pronounce it. Then read the dictionary meaning and pronunciation of the word, noting both in the margin of your notes. Keep in mind that if the author used the word once, he'll probably use it again.

If the text contains a lot of difficult words, you may want to read through some of the material first, marking the difficult words or making a list of the words that need to be looked up. Then go back for a second pass with a dictionary close at hand.

It's especially important to understand the meaning of technical terms when reading scientific material. Technical terms are integral to understanding scientific principles being discussed. By building your vocabulary, you not only better understand the material, but also become better able to express yourself, both verbally and in writing.

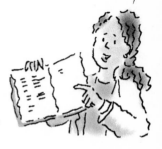

Well, I've marked all the difficult words I need to look up. That leaves and, but, the, and of.

Summarizing the material

In general, textbooks use the same method in every chapter to summarize the chapter's content. This information may be contained in a summary paragraph or a group of summary questions. After reading your assignment, look at the chapter summary and table of contents again to be sure you understood the material in the format intended by the author. If there's an area you're unsure of, read through that information again or ask for clarification from your instructor, who can probably explain it better.

Slow and steady

If you need to read the material again to understand it better, do it differently the second time. Read the material more slowly, perhaps, concentrating on one sentence at a time. Or, read the material aloud. Make sure you understand each sentence before moving to the next. Try to relate the new idea to what the author has already covered.

Can we talk?

After you've finished the assignment, find ways to apply your newly acquired knowledge, even if just by talking about it. Share what you read with others. Talking about the material reflects your ability to restate what you've learned, which reinforces your comprehension.

Increasing your reading rate

The average college student reads fiction and nontechnical materials at a rate of 250 to 350 words per minute. To reach peak efficiency in reading, experts say your reading speed should approach 500 to 700 words per minute. Some people can read at a rate of 1,000 words per minute or even faster.

Increasing the rate at which you read can help you move through assignments more quickly, thus improving your study efficiency. However, keep in mind that when it comes to reading speed, faster isn't better if you don't understand what you've read. The trick is to read faster *and* comprehend the material.

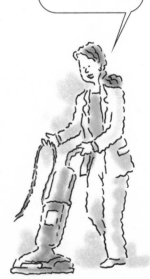

Faster is better only when you can understand the signs along the way.

Rapid eye movement

The key to rapid reading is to sweep your eyes from left to right across the page, making as few stops — called *fixations* — as possible. Readers who can see a full phrase at a time can read faster than those who see one word at a time.

When you read, your eyes tend to jump toward information you've already read. In some situations, you can spend as much as 90% of your reading time with your eyes looking away from what you think you're looking at. Training your eyes to reduce eye movement can double reading speed almost immediately.

When reading rapidly, it helps to sweep your eyes from left to right!

Optimum optics

To train your eyes to stay where you want them when reading, hold a blank index card above each line you read. As you progress down the page, use the card to cover each line after you've finished reading it. At first you might find this process physically different because your eyes naturally want to scan back up the page, but after a few weeks you'll find that you're reading faster than ever.

Role of speed in the reading process

Does reading faster compromise comprehension? Researchers say no, particularly if the technique used to improve the reading rate focuses on improving basic reading habits. Most adults are able to increase their rate of reading without lowering comprehension. In fact, an increase in rate is typically paralleled by an increase in comprehension. Furthermore, people who increase their reading speed don't understand material better if they slow down. So, reading faster is, in many instances, a win-win situation.

What's slowing you down?

A number of factors play a role in keeping the reading rate slower than it could be, including:

- reading word by word
- slow reaction time
- slow recognition and response to the material
- reading aloud
- faulty eye movements, including wrong placement on the page, faulty return sweep (movement from line to line), and irregular rhythm and movement
- habitual rereading
- inattention
- impaired retention
- lack of practice
- deliberate rate suppression out of fear of losing comprehension
- habitual slow reading
- poor differentiation between important aspects and those that can be safely skimmed over
- inability to remember critical details.

Preparing to increase your reading rate

Certain conditions should be met before trying to increase your reading rate:

- Have your eyes checked; slow reading is sometimes related to uncorrected vision defects. To ease eye strain and lessen eye movement while reading, hold your book 4″ to 6″ farther away from your eyes than you normally do. Be sure to hold reading material at least 15″ away from your eyes.
- Avoid sounding out words as you read. Reading silently is two to three times faster than reading aloud. Concentrate on key words and ideas rather than on whispering each word to yourself.
- Avoid rereading. Rereading is generally just a bad habit rather than a symptom of the need to improve comprehension. Many of the ideas that may need further explanation are explained later in the text. Slower readers tend to reread more often, possibly due to an inability to concentrate or a lack of confidence in their ability to comprehend the material.
- Develop a wider eye span by focusing on taking in more words on a line as you read. (See *Widening your eye span*, page 66.) Most people read one word at a time, but the brain can assimilate several words at once. Developing a wider eye span helps you reduce the number of reading stops, which, in turn, yields a faster reading rate.

> **Memory jogger**
>
> Play your **CARDs** right when increasing your reading rate. Remember to do these four key steps:
>
> **C**orrect vision problems.
>
> **A**void rereading.
>
> **R**ead silently.
>
> **D**evelop a wider eye span.

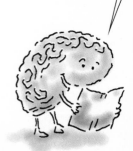

Want to get out of that one-word-at-a-time reading rut? Bring it on! I can assimilate several words at once.

Exercise your mind

Widening your eye span

Readers whose eyes take in more than one word at a time can read faster and retain just as much information as a reader whose eyes take in only one word at a time. Try this exercise to help you see the whole page rather than zooming in on single words. Perform this exercise 5 minutes per day, every day for several weeks. Use a large book when practicing.

1. Flip through the pages of the book quickly, turning them from the top with your left hand and scrolling left to right down each page with the edge of your right hand.

2. Follow your right hand down each page with your eyes, trying to see as many words as possible. Start by drifting down each page for 2 or 3 seconds, gradually reducing the time spent on each page until you can go as fast as you can turn pages.

3. Start by reading at a rate of 20 pages per minute. Slowly increase this rate over a period of 1 to 2 months to as many as 100 pages per minute.

Adjusting your reading rate

Your reading rate shouldn't be the same for all the material you read. Adjust your reading rate according to the difficulty level and the specific purpose for reading. Use a faster rate for easy, familiar, or interesting material, and a slower rate for unfamiliar content or language. (See *Calculating average reading speed.*) Keep in mind that as your vocabulary improves, so does your reading speed. The fewer stops you make to stumble over an unknown word, the faster you can move through the material.

What's your purpose?

Avoid planning to read your assignments at your maximum reading rate. Take into account those areas of the reading assignment that may be difficult to read as well as those that may be easier. Decide on your purpose in reading, and then read at a rate that best provides the level of comprehension you require.

Know when to slow down...

In general, you should slow your reading speed when you encounter:
• complex sentence or paragraph structure
• material that must be remembered in detail
• detailed or highly technical material, including complicated instructions and statements of difficult principles
• unfamiliar or unclear terminology (Try to understand the material in context, and then continue reading, returning to that section later.)
• unfamiliar or abstract concepts. (Try to internalize the information by making it applicable to your personal life.)

Advice from the experts

Calculating average reading speed

Use your average reading rate when planning your reading schedule. To figure your average reading rate, perform this calculation:

• Count the total number of words in 10 lines of text. Divide this figure by 10 to get the average number of words per line.

• Count the total number of lines on a full page of text.

• Multiply the average number of words per line by the number of lines on a page. This is the *word density* of the material. Keep in mind that word density can vary from book to book.

• Read for exactly 10 minutes. (Time yourself.)

• Multiply the number of pages read in 10 minutes by the word density to get an approximate number of words read.

• Divide the total number of words read by 10 (the number of minutes read). This is your *reading rate* for this text.

Sample calculation

Here's a sample calculation of a person's average reading speed for a textbook that consists of about 125 words in 10 lines and holds 52 lines on each page.

$$\frac{125 \text{ words}}{10 \text{ lines}} = 12.5 \text{ words/line}$$

$$52 \text{ lines/page} \times 12.5 \text{ words/line} = 650 \text{ words/page}$$

$$\frac{650 \text{ words/page} \times 3.5 \text{ pages read in 10 minutes}}{10 \text{ minutes}} = 227.5 \text{ words/minute}$$

...and when to speed up

In general, accelerate your reading speed when you encounter:

• simple material that contains few new ideas

• broad or generalized ideas or statements of ideas already explained

• detailed explanations and elaborations of ideas that aren't necessary for your purpose

• examples and illustrations that cover material you already understand. (Examples and illustrations are included in the text to clarify ideas, but they become unnecessary if you already know the material.)

So many words, so little time

Of the more than 600,000 words in the English language, 400 of them are used over and over again in most of the material you'll ever read. These 400 words, called *structure words*, make up 65% of printed works. Structure words include such words as *the*, *and*, *to*, *from*, *but*, and *however*. Even though you shouldn't completely skip words in a sentence, you shouldn't stop on structure words either. Let your eye take them in along with neighboring words to speed reading along.

Practice, practice, practice

As you practice reading faster, you'll become more adept at it. However, always read all of the words in a passage; otherwise, you may misinterpret the author's meaning or miss a relevant point. In addition, reading faster than you can understand the material can provoke frustration and anxiety.

If you're concerned that reading faster will make you miss words, remember that practice makes perfect — or at least better. You may also find it helpful to visualize yourself as an improved, faster reader. Visualizing yourself as you would like to be can help you attain your goal.

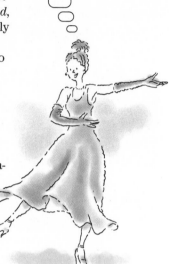

I visualize myself as a really great dancer...

Basic classroom skills

The instructor's goal in giving a lecture is to make the content easier to understand. The instructor includes explanations and clarifies ideas and information included in your textbook. To improve your ability to retain information provided in the classroom, you'll need to take specific steps before and during class and to organize your notes and other class materials for maximum efficiency.

Preparing for class

To prepare properly for a lecture, look at the reading assignment. Use the skimming techniques you learned at the beginning of this chapter.

First things first

Read the section headings. Then look at charts or illustrations in the chapter, and read the captions for each. Skim the main text to identify basic concepts and the most important information. Look for words emphasized in boldface or italics print.

At this point, your goal is to gain a general understanding of the content. Try not to get bogged down in difficult sections; the lecture may clarify those sections for you.

Write questions that come to mind as you read, but keep the questions brief — most of them will probably be answered during the lecture. If they aren't, you'll be better prepared to ask the instructor for clarification.

A second look

After you finish your first reading, look again at the headings and illustrations. This quick review increases your long-term memory and allows you to more effectively integrate what you learn in class with what you read before class.

Classroom learning

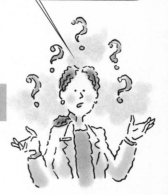

Have questions? Jot them down as they come to mind, and you'll be ready to ask them in class.

During class, pay special attention to:
• contents of handouts
• anything written on the board
• anything the instructor stresses or repeats
• the instructor's response to questions from classmates
• your own thoughts, questions, or reactions to lecture material
• anything the instructor takes a long time to explain
• anything discussed that isn't covered in the textbook, particularly the instructor's personal views
• how the instructor presents the information — for instance, whether she presents the "big picture" or the details
• the beginning and end of the lecture. Instructors commonly summarize their entire lecture during the first few minutes; in the last few minutes, they summarize major points and other important points that weren't covered earlier.

Learning from lectures

In a lecture, communication takes place primarily between the instructor and the students. How well you listen to your instructor depends on your background knowledge, the difficulty of the concepts being covered, and your purpose for listening. (See *Levels of listening*, page 70.)

How well you listen may also be affected by the instructor's teaching style. For most students, listening to lectures is a passive activity — but it doesn't have to be. Try to stay involved in the lecture, thinking of questions as the speaker lectures. Jot down a key word or two about each question in the margin of your notes. Then, when the instructor asks whether anyone has questions, refer to your notes to ask the questions you raised earlier.

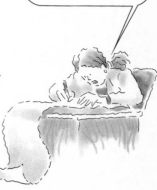

Heads up! Don't bury your face in your hands. Keep an eye on your instructor to see what material she considers most important.

Levels of listening

Listening occurs on several levels, depending on the effort expended by the listener. This chart describes the different levels of listening.

Level	Description
Reception	Hearing without thought
Attention	Listening passively; no effort to understand what's being said
Definition	Lowest level of active listening; giving meaning to isolated facts and details; no overall organizational plan
Integration	Relating new information to old learning
Interpretation	Synthesizing information; putting information into your own words
Implication	Drawing conclusions
Application	Applying information to personal experience; using information in new situations
Evaluation	Judging information in terms of accuracy and relevance

Slow down — you move too fast!

When the instructor seems to run through a lecture quickly, covering a lot of material in a limited time, it may be wise to interrupt and ask for clarification, particularly if you familiarized yourself with the material beforehand but still don't understand it. When asking for clarification, be as specific as possible. Try to show that you understood some of what was said by rephrasing the information in your own words.

Pick up the pace

Daydreaming is more likely to be a problem when a class is slow. To stave off boredom and loss of concentration, try to rephrase, repeat, and apply what has been said. Use slow parts of the class to review material in your head. Review concepts and definitions that the instructor has introduced and try rephrasing them in your own words. Then repeat new phrases and definitions to yourself and try to memorize them. Or, try to anticipate the instructor's next move. This keeps you involved in the class and trains you to follow the instructor's thought processes, which helps you to perform better on assignments.

In too deep?

If you aren't understanding the material well, you may not have the background that other students in the class have. The feeling of being lost usually comes from the lack of a sufficient foundation of knowledge in a particular area. In each class, the instructor assumes a certain amount of knowledge on the part of the students, and tries to build on that knowledge.

If that foundation doesn't exist, it's easy to tune out what the instructor is saying. Instead of tuning out the instructor, focus on tuning in even more carefully. Keep taking notes even though you don't comprehend everything. Jot down words and phrases that you don't understand. Look them up right after the class, or ask the instructor for clarification.

Keeping the lines open

Maintaining communication between you and your instructor can help her clarify points of misunderstanding. In addition, your respectful feedback can help reinforce the instructor's method or point out places a lecture may be weak.

If it's a bore, try not to snore

Contrary to popular opinion, your instructor is actually a human being! She may be brilliant in her field, but that's no guarantee that she's equally brilliant at communicating all the facts, ideas, and concepts she wants her students to learn.

You may need to compensate for a less effective speaker by defining, integrating, and interpreting information and drawing conclusions for yourself. (See *Compensating for an ineffective lecturer*, page 72.) Finding ways to apply information and judge its value then becomes one of your primary jobs.

In a lecture, the speaker controls what information is conveyed to the class. Your job is to determine what the instructor expects and to keep that purpose in mind while listening and reacting to the lecture. To help you maintain active listening during a lecture, follow these steps:

• Keep your purpose for listening in mind.
• Pay careful attention to the instructor's introductory and summary statements, which usually state main points.
• Continue to take notes.
• Sit comfortably erect to convey your interest and stave off sleepiness.
• Keep your eyes on the instructor.
• Concentrate on what the instructor is saying to ignore external distractions and eliminate internal ones.
• Question the material.
• Listen for transition words that signal main points.

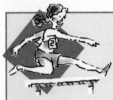

Overcoming obstacles

Compensating for an ineffective lecturer

Does this student's problem sound familiar? Read and learn.

Question

I'm taking a course, and the instructor isn't a very good lecturer. I'm having a hard time understanding, and I'm getting frustrated. Do you have any tips?

Words of wisdom

Your main task when faced with any lecturer is to get the most out of the class regardless of the lecturer's effectiveness. When a lecturer isn't effective, you can still obtain the knowledge you need by following a few guidelines. This chart explains what to do when an instructor falls short of expectations.

If your instructor fails to do this	Then you do this
Explain goals of the lecture	Use your text and syllabus to set objectives.
Review previous lecture material before beginning a new lecture	Set aside time before each class to review notes.
State main ideas in an introduction and summary of the lecture	Write short summaries of the day's lecture immediately after class.
Provide an outline of the lecture	Preview assigned readings before class, or outline notes after class.
Provide "wait time" for writing notes	Politely ask the instructor to repeat information or to speak more slowly.
Speak clearly with appropriate volume	Politely ask the instructor to repeat information or to speak louder, or move closer to her.
Answer questions without sarcasm	Refrain from taking comments personally.
Stay on topic	Discover how anecdotes relate to the topic, or use anecdotes as a memory cue.

If your instructor fails to do this	Then you do this
Refrain from reading directly from the text	Mark passages in text as the instructor reads, or summarize or outline these passages in the text margin.
Emphasize main points	Supplement lectures through text previews and reading.
Use transition words	Supplement notes with terms listed in the text, and highlight information contained in the lecture.
Give examples to illustrate difficult ideas	Ask the instructor for a clarifying example, discuss idea with other students, or create an example yourself.
Write important words, dates, and other key information on the board	Use the text glossary or a dictionary.
Define important terms	Relate information to what you know about the topic, or create a clarifying example for yourself.

- Mark words or references you don't understand for later investigation.
- Adjust your listening and note-taking pace to the lecture.
- Avoid being a distraction yourself by sitting still and remaining silent.

Active listening

Active listening occurs when you consciously think about how you're listening and use strategies to improve and maximize your listening skills. To improve your active listening skills, you need to:

- avoid behaviors that can interfere with listening
- recognize main ideas
- use transition cues effectively
- differentiate more important information from less important information.

Do not disturb

A number of behaviors can interfere with your understanding when listening to a lecturer or other speaker, including:

- allowing yourself to be distracted
- zoning out when difficult material is presented
- becoming overexcited by something in the lecture
- considering the subject uninteresting
- criticizing the speaker's delivery or mannerisms
- daydreaming
- faking attentiveness
- letting emotion-laden words arouse personal antagonism
- listening primarily for facts instead of ideas
- trying to outline everything.

Heads up!

Every lecture is structured to center around main ideas. This structure leads to certain patterns that vary with the instructor's purposes. Be aware that in a lecture an instructor may:

- introduce new topics or summarize information
- list or rank details
- present opposing sides of an issue
- identify causes and effects or problems and solutions
- discuss concepts using supporting details.

Take the hint

Signal words and other verbal markers help you identify and anticipate the flow of a lecture. Becoming familiar with *transition words* helps you organize lecture notes and listen more actively.

For example, the word *conversely* probably indicates that the lecturer is about to present an opposing point of view. *Therefore* means the lecturer is summing up cause and effect. *Finally* means the instructor is getting to the end of her point or series of points.

Identifying important information

Your ability to identify important information contributes to your ability to become a more active listener. Although instructors emphasize main points differently, they have similar ways of conveying important information. Some instructors, for instance, write key information on the board or present the information using a PowerPoint slide show. PowerPoint presentations allow instructors to present the information visually with an accompanying outline for note-taking.

Other instructors outline the entire lecture on the board before class begins. Some write key points or terms on the board as they lecture.

Be a copycat

Copying outlines or lists of terms from the board aids learning in three ways. First, you learn as you write. Copying the outline also provides a nutshell view of the lecture's content and serves as a guide for later study.

Instructors also convey information by:
• pausing, which gives you more time to take comprehensive notes
• repeating information
• changing the tone or volume of their voices to make a point
• telling the class what's worth remembering for a test
• using body language (If your instructor gestures to stress a point, it's often an essential point for you to understand.)
• using visual aids (The use of films, overhead transparencies, videotapes, and other audiovisual materials signals important topics.)
• referring to specific text pages. (Information an instructor knows by page number is worth noting and remembering.)

Listen with LISAN

Active listening is the key to taking notes during a lecture. The *LISAN method* of taking notes encourages active listening and can improve understanding and retention. The LISAN method involves these guidelines:
• **L**ead; don't follow. Anticipate what the instructor is going to say.
• **I**deas. What's the main idea?
• **S**ignal words. Listen for words that indicate the direction the instructor is taking.
• **A**ctively listen. Ask questions, be prepared.
• **N**ote-taking. Write down key points; be selective.

Developing learning skills

You can also develop your learning skills as you listen. Developing these skills involves memorizing, applying knowledge, interpreting information, and recognizing shifts in teaching styles.

Is it live, or is it memorized?

Introductory courses tend to demand a lot of memorization. Stay alert for information you should commit to memory. Such pieces of information as phrases, dates, and diagrams written on the board are probably items that the instructor expects you to remember. If the instructor takes the time to write a definition or prepare a handout or slide, that means the information is important and should be remembered. If the instructor speaks more slowly than usual or repeats information, she's probably giving you time to take notes on the material.

How can I apply it? Let me count the ways

Many instructors arrange their classes and assignments to encourage you to apply the information they provide to clinical situations. Pay attention to how the instructor structures the class. For instance, if the instructor gives written assignments on the material, you'll need to show in writing how well you can apply your new knowledge.

Does the instructor spend class time working through problems or cases? If so, you'll probably be expected to know how to work through such problems on a test. Does the instructor ask students to solve problems at the board? If so, expect to be asked to demonstrate your new knowledge in a clinical situation.

Hmmm, how should I interpret that?

Many advanced science and health classes require that students use their interpretative skills. The instructor tries to foster development of those skills by asking a lot of general questions and offering guidance. In these kinds of classes, the students do most of the talking, and the assignments tend to consist primarily of reading and observing.

Heed the clues

Be on the lookout for shifts in teaching style. For example, if an instructor stops a class discussion to write dates on the board, she has switched from an interpretive mode to a memorization mode. Write down the dates. Some instructors give obvious clues to what's important to study—for example, by saying something as clear and simple as "This is important."

Psychology 101

Other clues aren't as obvious. Look for patterns in behavior, such as an instructor who gets up and paces whenever she begins warming up to an important point. The more attuned you are to the instructor's behaviors, the more knowledge you can gain from the material being presented.

> Computer-assisted instruction can be a boon to students with families and full-time jobs.

Computer-assisted instruction

Learning by computer, or *computer-assisted instruction (CAI)*, has become popular in the last few years to help fulfill a variety of educational goals. The most effective CAI programs require only basic computer skills. Many CAI applications combine a variety of formats to offer the student various ways to learn. Common CAI formats include:

- drill and practice
- tutorial
- simulation
- computer-managed instruction
- problem solving.

Repeat and improve

Drill-and-practice software allows learners to master facts, relationships, problems, and vocabulary. The software usually offers groups of questions with similar content, which allows the student to hone specific skills. The software may be designed to offer more difficult questions as the student progresses through the application.

Tutor in a box

Tutorial software aims to teach concepts rather than allow the practice of individual skills. This software presents concepts in several formats, including text and images, and commonly incorporates feedback to student responses. Tutorials may employ pretesting or posttesting to instruct students at the appropriate teaching level.

Simulated scenarios

A *simulation* is a computer-generated visual and auditory experience. Computer simulations allow students to experience real-life events in the safety of the classroom. Because simulations usually demand decision-making skills, the student becomes directly involved in the outcomes.

Computer in charge

Computer-managed instruction assesses the knowledge level and educational goals of students. Through computerized testing, this software can help instructors assess students and design a curriculum to fit students' needs.

Time to apply

Problem-solving software is useful after students become familiar with basic necessary concepts. Problem-solving software can then help students use those concepts to solve difficult problems and advance their level of thinking.

Organizing lecture content

Lectures can be *text-dependent,* meaning that they follow the organization of the text closely, or *text-independent,* in which other media are used to enhance the delivery of information.

Lectures by the book

During a text-dependent lecture, write notes and instructions emphasized during the lecture directly in your textbook, highlighting or underlining as the instructor speaks. This is an especially helpful technique if you read the text before class. You can also cross out information your instructor says is unnecessary and note important information in the margins of the chapter and in your notebook.

Working without backup

When lectures are independent of the text, they're based on what the instructor thinks is most important about the topic. In those instances, your responsibility for taking notes increases. Because you don't have the text to use as a backup source, review or outline the lecture soon after class to give it some form of organization. Discuss your notes with other students, or augment the lecture with supplemental reading. Set some study objectives to help you create a purpose for learning and increase your recall.

Stimulating the senses

Instructors use a variety of media — handouts, illustrations, PowerPoint presentations, videos or DVDs, models, and more — to stimulate students' senses during lectures. Media and advancing technology offer visually interesting ways to add knowledge and information, arouse emotion or interest, and increase skills and performance.

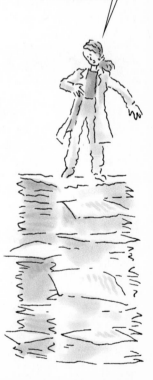

I sure do take more notes when lectures are independent of text material. Wow!

When an instructor creates or chooses the medium to be used, the information it contains tends to be course-specific and corresponds closely to what the instructor expects you to know.

Your responsibility is to recognize your instructor's purposes for using each particular medium, and judge its worth in meeting your learning needs. For example, if you have extensive knowledge of a topic, a film about that topic may serve only as a review. If the topic is new to you, the same film may be aimed at building background knowledge.

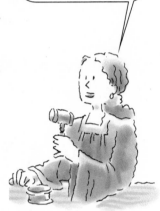

You be the judge! It's your responsibility to determine why your instructor uses a particular medium and to render a verdict on how well that medium meets your learning needs!

Student-teacher conferences

Whenever you have questions about the content discussed in class, the instructor's expectations of you as a learner, or other important aspects of a course, you may want to set up a conference with the instructor. Before the conference, make sure you have a specific topic of discussion in mind. Your first test may make an ideal subject, particularly if you feel as if you're struggling with the course material.

Having a conference with your instructor helps you understand the instructor better. It also lets you demonstrate your interest in improving your performance. Even if you think you're doing well in a class, meeting with the instructor can help ensure that your perception is accurate, and can help you establish rapport.

Effective note-taking skills

Taking notes may be the most crucial part of active listening during lectures. In your effort to capture everything significant said by the instructor, you'll not only need to use all of your listening ability and concentration during the lecture, but you'll also need a good system for recording what was said. Taking effective notes involves understanding why you take notes in the first place and following some practical guidelines for taking them.

Usefulness of notes

Notes commonly trigger your memory of the lecture or the text. In general, students who review notes achieve more than those who don't. Researchers have found that if important information was contained in notes, students tended to remember that information 34% of the time. Information not found in notes was remembered only 5% of the time. Even if you understand your instructor's lecture fully and have no questions, take notes anyway. Later, you'll want to know what the instructor thought was important, and you'll use the notes to refresh your memory.

Listen up!

Taking notes also makes you pay more attention to the new material, thereby allowing you to become more familiar with it. Note-taking requires more effort than reading and therefore requires you to take an active role in class. By paraphrasing and condensing information as you take notes, you show your understanding of the information and your ability to relate the information to your background knowledge.

Tips for taking notes

To take effective notes, you'll need to use your own form of note-taking shorthand, organize your notes after class, keep your notes personal, avoid using a tape recorder, and employ other note-taking strategies.

Shrthnd spds note tkng

Taking notes rapidly involves doing as little writing as possible while capturing all of the facts, principles, and ideas expressed by the lecturer. Fast note-taking can be enhanced by:
• abbreviating common words consistently (See *Common note-taking abbreviations and symbols*, page 80.)
• leaving out conjunctions, prepositions, and other words not essential to understanding a thought
• thinking before you write (but without thinking so long that you fall behind)
• creating a shorthand word or symbol for something used repeatedly in a lecture (for example, abbreviating systolic blood pressure as *SBP* in a discussion about hypertension)
• marking for emphasis, such as through the use of asterisks, exclamation points, underlining, color coding, or highlighting
• using shapes or varying handwriting size to stay organized. (You're more likely to recall information supplemented with visual clues, such as geometric shapes or different-sized handwriting.)

Postclass organization

After class, organize your notes. Write down the date at the beginning of each lecture, and number the pages so you can keep track of what you're doing. Make a note of your assignments, what they involve, and when they're due.

Keep 'em personal

The most effective notes are personal, reflecting the note-taker's background knowledge and understanding. Borrowed or bought

Memory jogger

Remember the mnemonic **CATTLE** when taking effective notes:

Create a shorthand for repeated words.

Abbreviate common words.

Think before writing.

Try using shapes or varying handwriting.

Leave out unessential words.

Emphasize important words or topics.

Advice from the experts

Common note-taking abbreviations and symbols

To speed note taking, get in the habit of using abbreviations and symbols. This chart lists common abbreviations and symbols used for taking notes.

Abbreviations		Symbols	
abt	about	®	right
b/c	because	Ⓛ	left
dx	diagnose or diagnosis	↑	increase, increased, or increasing
e.g.	for example	↓	decrease, decreased, or decreasing
h/a	headache	→	leads to or causes
hx	history	>	more than
imp	important	<	less than
incl	including	Δ	change
pt	patient	~	about, approximately
px	physical	+	and, in addition
rx	treat or treatment	#	pounds or number
s/e	side effects	☆	important or stressed by instructor
s/s	signs and symptoms	p̄	after
w/	with	ā	before
w/o	without	–	negative
		c̄	with
		s̄	without

notes require no effort or action on the part of the learner; thus they do little to help the student learn. To get the most out of notes for a class, make sure you attend the class yourself and take your own notes.

Borrowed notes do have a place, however, when they're all that's available. If you've been absent from class, you may have no choice but to borrow someone else's notes.

Taping is a sticky business

Tape-recording a lecture can be useful, but only if you also take notes during the lecture, allowing the taped material to pick up any important points you miss. If you can't attend a class, asking a classmate to audiotape the class may prove the next-best thing to being there. Otherwise, using a tape recorder to record lectures is probably not a good idea. Here's why:

• Listening to the tape takes as long as, if not longer than, listening to the lecture itself.

• To record the main ideas and highlights of the lecture, you have to make notes from the tape, which takes even longer.
• Taped material doesn't reflect diagrams or additional written material the instructor may have used during the class.
• Technical difficulties, such as a flawed tape or a dead battery, sometimes arise, causing you to miss part or all of a lecture.
• Some instructors may not allow tape-recorder use. Ask the instructor before class whether it's permissible to record a lecture.

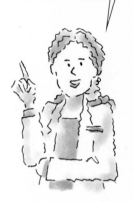

Take notes even if you disagree with what the instructor says.

Other note-taking strategies

Most students take reasonably good notes but then don't use them properly. They tend to wait until just before an examination to review their notes; by then, the notes have lost much of their meaning. Remember that active listening and note-taking go hand in hand. To help you keep your notes specific, organized, and comprehensive, follow these pointers:
• Even if you disagree with a point being made by the instructor, write it down.
• Raise questions whenever appropriate.
• Develop and use a standard method of note-taking, including punctuation and abbreviations.
• Keep notes in a large, loose-leaf binder, which allows you to more easily use an outline form for your notes. The binder also allows you to reorganize your notes easily when preparing for a test or quiz. (See *Cornell system of note-taking*, page 82.)
• Leave a few spaces blank as the lecture progresses, so that additional points can be filled in later.
• Don't write down every word the lecturer says. Spend more time listening; try to write down the main points, but know that sometimes it's more important to think than to write.
• Listen for transition cues, such as a change in vocal inflection, that signify important points or a transition from one point to the next.
• Make your original notes legible enough for you to read later.
• Copy everything your instructor writes on the board. You may not be able to integrate the information with your lecture notes, but you'll have the information in your notes for later referral.
• Sit at the front of the class, where there are fewer distractions.

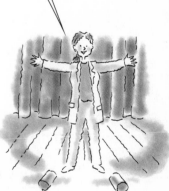

If the theatrics of film and television distract you from note-taking during class, take notes after the "show," or ask to see it again.

That's entertainment

Taking notes from films, slides, or television differs from traditional note-taking because these types of media are associated with entertainment. As a result, you may not realize the importance of the information they provide. Furthermore,

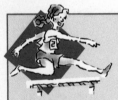

Overcoming obstacles

Cornell system of note-taking

Are your notes a mess like this student's? Look over her shoulder for some words of wisdom.

Question

My instructor doesn't use a PowerPoint slide show to present new information. After class, I look at my notes and they're a mess. How can I take better notes?

Words of wisdom

The *Cornell system* can help you develop organized notes. Before the lecture, obtain a large, loose-leaf binder. Use only one side of the paper. Divide your paper as shown in the illustration at right.

During the lecture

Use the "Notes" area on the right side of the page to take notes in paragraph form. Capture general ideas, not illustrative ideas. Skip a line to show the end of an idea or thought. Use abbreviations whenever possible to save time. Write legibly.

After the lecture

Read through your notes and make them more legible as needed. Use the "Cue" column to jot down ideas or key words that highlight the main aspects of the lecture. Cover the "Notes" area with a blank piece of paper and describe the general ideas and concepts of the lecture using the notes in the "Cue" column. Use the "Summary" area to summarize your notes in one or two sentences.

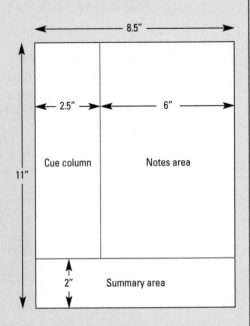

these types of media are usually shown in a darkened room, which is hardly conducive to note-taking.

The fast pace of these formats is another stumbling block to note-taking. A film or television show doesn't provide many pauses for taking notes. For this reason, taking notes immediately after the presentation is sometimes the best alternative for recording new information. If a presentation was on film or slides, ask whether you can watch the presentation again or check to see if the instructor puts the presentation on reserve in the library.

Take a note on note-taking outlines

Making a *note-taking outline* before the lecture gives you a basis for understanding the lecture and a chance to locate important terms, concepts, and dates beforehand. To construct a note-taking outline, divide each page of notes vertically into two sections, with one-third of the space to the left and two-thirds to the right. Then record the chapter title and major and minor headings on the left side, estimating the amount of space that each section may require.

When previewing the material, survey the physical characteristics of the chapter, including length, text structure, visual aids, and term identification. Read the chapter introduction or first paragraph. Survey graphs, maps, charts, and diagrams. Look for such typographic aids as **boldface,** <u>underlining</u>, and *italics*, used to highlight important new terms or ideas. Record the terms in the outline. Lastly, read the last paragraph or summary, which generally reviews the main points or conclusions of the chapter.

I'll note it myyyy way

Develop a system for taking notes that best fits your learning style and course content. Date each day's notes to serve as a reference point if you need to compare notes with someone else's or ask your instructor for clarification. If you're absent, the missing dates identify which notes you need. Other steps to personalizing your notes include:
• keeping your notes together in a notebook, preferably one with pockets that can be used to save class handouts
• bringing all necessary note-taking materials to each class
• knowing how to interpret your own shorthand
• grouping and labeling information to aid recall
• writing down facts and diagrams written on the board
• leaving room in your notes to fill in later
• skipping lines to separate important groups of ideas and writing on only one side of the paper, both of which will make it easier to read your notes later
• keeping your notes neat and your writing legible so you can read your own writing later
• organizing your notes after class
• using color coding to mark important ideas and concepts
• reading over your notes as soon as possible after class, while the material is still fresh in your mind, and correcting your notes as needed
• refraining from rewriting the text verbatim. If the instructor refers to a specific text page, go to the book and mark the information there. Remember to jot the page number in your notes and to write a brief summary later.

How much is enough?

How many notes are enough? That depends on your own confidence and your instructor's teaching style. Notes must be accurate and useful for refreshing your memory on important points.

You're probably making too few notes if you simply write down a list of facts without tying them together. Conversely, if you spend all your time writing notes, you don't have time to think about or question the material. Furthermore, you may miss an important point while writing down something less significant. Try to find an effective medium.

Style is everything

Be flexible enough to adapt your note-taking style to best fit the style of the instructor. One format for note-taking may work well for one instructor but not for another. Some possible note formats follow:

• *Outline.* If the lecture is highly organized, an outline will probably work well. Mark main section headings with uppercase roman numerals. Mark important points under each section with capital letters and supporting points under the important points with Arabic (regular) numerals. Subordinate sets of ideas can be indented and bulleted beneath the preceding higher level.

• *Thin-fat columns.* On your note paper, draw one thin column and one fat column. Use the thin column to keep track of extra notes to yourself, such as "See page 53 of text" or "Test on Tuesday." Also use this column for important facts to remember. Use the fat column to record lecture notes.

• *Equal columns.* Divide your note paper into two equal columns when comparing two concepts. Put notes about one concept on one side and notes about the other on the opposite side. You'll then have information about both concepts in addition to a visual way to compare and contrast the concepts.

• *Idea tree.* Start with the main idea circled in the center of the writing, and then branch off facts like branches from the tree. Branch off subordinate ideas like twigs branching off of larger branches. This format is also called *concept mapping*.

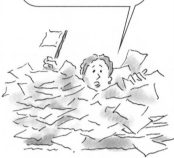

Don't overdo it. When it comes to note-taking, a happy medium will keep you from drowning in paperwork and missing the point!

Reviewing notes

After class, review your notes for clarity. Rewrite anything you think you may not be able to read later, particularly if you've used many abbreviations in your notes. Finish up open-ended notes that you didn't finish before moving on to the next topic.

Reviewing class notes can be particularly important after a disorganized lecture or one in which the instructor stated certain intentions at the beginning of the lecture but never fulfilled them. Reviewing these notes may take time and research because you may need to fill in blank spots with material from the textbook.

Reviewing your notes within 24 hours after taking them can help establish the information in your memory. If you

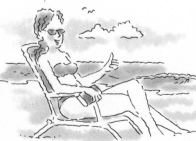

No, I'm not slacking off! I reviewed my notes a few hours after class, so now it's time to relax.

don't look over your notes within a day, they may not make sense anymore. In addition, read your notes again before the next class to give yourself a sense of continuity.

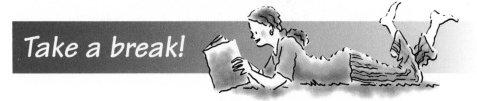

Take a break!

Term searching

Take a break from your reading material and find these 20 terms that help your reading and classroom strategies. Hint: Go up, down, across, and diagonal! The answers are on the next page.

D	F	N	O	R	B	A	E	R	G	T	S	S	O	R	T	E	N
R	E	S	K	I	M	M	I	N	G	G	O	H	L	M	M	Y	E
A	I	H	W	L	P	P	L	H	O	O	W	O	L	T	B	E	B
H	K	O	F	E	R	U	L	A	J	E	A	R	D	S	E	S	H
X	E	R	A	L	E	W	E	G	T	E	X	T	A	L	R	P	I
C	Y	T	Q	K	P	P	D	A	Q	U	A	R	Z	B	A	A	O
O	V	H	U	J	A	R	I	W	P	R	E	O	N	E	P	N	E
M	Y	A	G	Y	R	V	C	N	T	R	L	O	L	A	I	P	N
P	A	N	J	W	E	A	T	E	G	E	B	B	O	O	D	O	T
R	N	D	E	R	A	I	I	D	E	V	X	T	K	L	E	H	L
E	E	L	B	E	I	N	O	T	S	I	N	T	R	A	Y	G	I
H	R	B	O	V	L	A	N	O	T	E	S	S	B	M	E	D	S
E	A	B	E	E	I	R	A	Y	A	W	R	I	O	O	M	S	T
N	U	H	G	V	P	G	R	G	X	B	O	O	U	T	O	I	E
S	Y	C	R	I	H	R	Y	N	E	V	R	N	T	A	V	K	N
I	M	L	A	E	N	N	E	I	Y	S	C	A	L	C	E	E	I
O	V	A	T	W	A	M	A	D	S	O	M	S	I	A	M	L	N
N	C	R	S	A	E	Y	R	A	C	T	H	E	N	M	E	E	G
S	I	I	C	O	H	T	L	E	C	T	U	R	E	S	N	A	H
G	M	T	P	O	T	C	R	R	G	I	N	I	O	N	T	R	A
A	A	Y	O	D	L	A	E	R	G	B	V	E	I	R	T	O	N
I	Z	S	D	T	O	U	H	N	F	T	A	Y	O	T	N	H	S
F	G	S	Y	S	T	E	M	A	W	G	H	I	O	R	T	S	S
D	N	A	N	D	R	A	H	N	N	E	V	M	A	O	Z	J	O
Q	U	S	C	W	I	A	S	E	S	V	U	N	M	U	I	N	G

Abbreviate
Clarity
Classroom
Columns
Comprehension
Dictionary
Eye span
Lectures
Listening
Notes
Outline
Prepare
Rapid eye movement
Reading
Review
Shorthand
Skimming
Sweeping
System
Textbook

Answer key

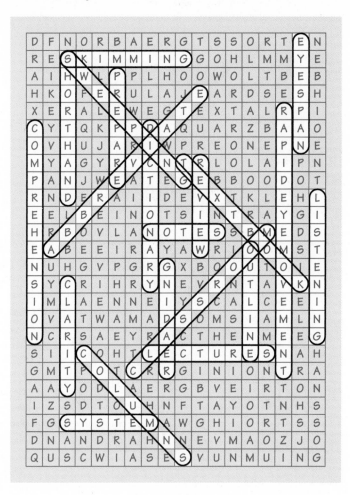

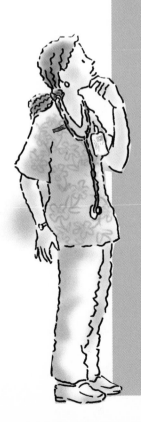

Part II How to take a test

Tips on test-taking

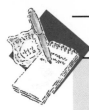

Just the facts

In this chapter, you'll learn:

♦ how to prepare mentally for a test, including how to construct a study plan, relax, and develop a positive attitude

♦ how to prepare physically for a test

♦ how objective examinations focus on recalling specific information

♦ how subjective examinations focus on your ability to explain ideas

♦ how learning about the results of a test can help you prepare for future tests.

Preparing for a test

Being a top test-taker demands preparation. The first step in that preparation is to recognize elements of test-related anxiety that may be preventing you from reaching your optimum performance level. After you've identified test anxiety elements, you can prepare your mind and body for the test.

Recognizing test anxiety

Test anxiety comes in many forms and may occur before the test or during the test itself. Types of test anxiety include:
• freezing up, in which your brain doesn't register the meaning of questions or you have to read test questions several times to comprehend them
• panicking about a difficult question or the thought of time running out
• worrying about the test

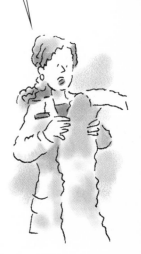

OK. I've identified my test anxiety elements (most of them, at least), so now I can prepare my mind and body for the big exam.

• being easily distracted, or spending time daydreaming about ways to escape rather than completing the test itself
• feeling nervous, which can prevent you from putting in the time necessary to succeed
• experiencing physical effects, such as nausea, muscle tension, headache, and sweating
• feeling a lack of interest in the test or topic. Some students find it easier not to care than to face their anxiety about performing well.

A little is OK

Feeling slightly anxious — but not *too* anxious — can improve your mental clarity and provide greater focus. Complacency, on the other hand, is more likely to result in falling short of your goals. If you find that you're consistently underperforming or feeling the physical effects of test anxiety — such as exhaustion, vague discomfort, and an inability to remember information — test anxiety may be getting the best of you.

I'm relaxed, and I will ace my test.
I'm relaxed, and I will pass my test.
I'm relaxed, and I will live through my test.

Preparing the mind

Most successful students use a combination of techniques to prepare themselves mentally to perform well on tests. To cope with test anxiety, you need to study well, relax, stay positive, and take well-planned breaks.

Anxiety antidote

Studying well can be the best antidote for test anxiety. The feeling of accomplishment that comes with an effective study regimen can banish many of the fears that cause test anxiety.

I've got rhythm, I've got clarity

Relaxation and other stress-reduction techniques can reduce test anxiety and give you the clarity of mind necessary to study effectively. Rhythmic breathing and meditation are two of the many techniques you may consider to reduce test anxiety.

Accentuate the positive

Test anxiety commonly stems from low self-esteem. Make an effort to think positively about the test experience. Tell yourself, "I can do it!" You'll be amazed how often positive results follow positive thinking.

I know I can, I know I can! You'd be surprised how much a little positive thinking can do to relieve test anxiety.

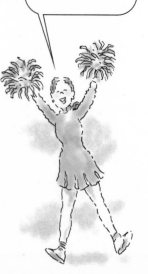

Take a breather!

Mild, short-term test anxiety can commonly be reduced by taking a short break. If you feel anxious during a test, sharpen your pencil or get a drink of water. If you feel anxious while studying, give yourself a quick break away from studying. Sometimes anxiety is your body's way of saying, "I need a few minutes off."

Preparing the body

Many students, even those with rigorous study habits, neglect their bodies when preparing for a test. Maximum test performance depends on meeting the need for proper rest, nutrition, and overall health. Physical preparedness is basic to improving your test-taking skills.

R and R

Rest and relaxation can overcome fatigue after intense mental or physical exertion. You can accomplish more when you feel rested and relaxed than when you're fatigued. To make sure you get enough rest and relaxation:
• get a sufficient amount of sleep
• change activities periodically
• exercise regularly
• relax periodically by watching television, listening to music, talking to friends, or reading a book (other than your textbook).

Mom was right!

Your posture during studying and examinations can affect your mood. Slouching not only hurts your back but also can make you feel sluggish and uninterested. Maintain good posture, and watch your focus improve.

Feed your brain

Because nutrition affects your physical well-being, it also affects your study habits and test-taking skills. Because class time, work time, and study time may conflict with eating on a regular schedule, counterbalance odd mealtimes with nutritious snacks or meals. Avoid excessive intake of caffeine or sugar, because these substances will cause your energy level to peak and trough.

Fever procedure

Even when you're in strong physical condition, you may become too ill to study properly to take a test. Don't neglect symptoms of illness in favor of studying for an upcoming test; you'll most likely feel ill during the test and, as a result, perform poorly. If you become ill, contact the instructor as soon as possible. This commu-

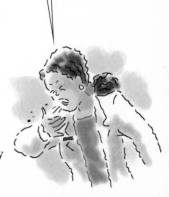

Don't be a hero. If you're sick, contact your instructor about rescheduling your test, and take your doctor's advice.

nicates your concern about missing the test and helps alleviate your own anxiety about missing it. Follow all of your doctor's guidelines for getting well again, including taking medications as prescribed and resting as much as the doctor advises.

Healthy habits

When a test is coming up, don't do anything that will upset your sense of normalcy. If you normally walk 30 minutes each day after lunch, don't jog during that time to relieve stress; you'll probably end up being sore, tired, *and* stressed. If you normally sleep 8 hours per night, avoid pulling an all-nighter. You may end up throwing off your sleep pattern and becoming sleep-deprived — not a healthy state for your brain just before a test.

Planning for a test

Successful students think about upcoming tests long before the day of the examination. They learn all they can about the test itself and then construct their study time accordingly.

Learning about the test

Before studying for a test, find out what kind of test it's going to be. If you know what kind of test to expect, your studying time will be more focused. For *objective tests* (short-answer, sentence-completion, multiple-choice, matching, and true-false tests), focus your studying on knowing facts and details and being able to recognize related material. For *essay* or *oral tests*, preparation includes being able to argue persuasively about several general topics and being able to back up those arguments with details.

In any case, you'll need to find out key pieces of information about the test to prepare properly, including facts about the test format and objectives, the availability of past tests, and the overall structure of the class.

Size it up

To find out about a test, ask the instructor. Many instructors explain the format of their tests to the whole class. Others inform only those students who ask these questions. For the latter instructors especially, make sure to ask about test format. When faced with an upcoming test, ask:

• Will the test be comprehensive, or will it cover certain chapters only? (See *That wasn't in the book.*)
• How many questions will it contain?
• How will the questions be weighted?

> To get the 411 on an upcoming test, search for the clues. Ask the instructor, check out the library, and stake out the class for structure clues.

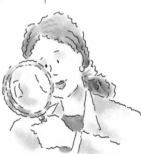

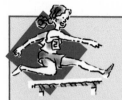

Overcoming obstacles

That wasn't in the book

Are you having trouble deciding what to study? Heed the advice that this student receives.

Question

It seems that there's always something on the test that wasn't covered in the textbook. So how do I prepare for the test?

Words of wisdom

Some instructors give their lecture material more weight than textbook material when composing test questions. Don't assume that a test will cover mostly information found in the textbook. Attempt to get the most from your lecture notes by considering these guidelines:

• Listen carefully to the instructor and take frequent notes.

• Try to identify what the instructor thinks is important, especially when she repeats or emphasizes information.

• Play an active role by digging deep into each lecture and applying the information to a real-life situation.

• Attend all lectures. If missing a lecture can't be avoided, get the class notes or PowerPoint presentation from a classmate.

• Sit in the front two or three rows so you can see and hear well.

• Will it be subjective or objective?
• Will it require that I apply knowledge or just know facts?
• How important is this test to my final grade?
• What can I bring to the test? Will calculators be allowed? Will formulas be supplied?
• Who is making the test?
• Who will grade the test?
• Will it be a special type of examination, such as a take-home test or an open-book test?

Look to the past

If you've previously taken tests in this course, you may already have an idea of what the upcoming test will be like. Past experience may tell you that the previous test focused on details rather than principles or that it contained an occasional "trick" question.

If this is your first test in the course, check for copies of past examinations. These may be available from the instructor or may be on file with the instructor's department or college library. Study the examinations for ideas about what to expect, but don't expect identical questions or directions.

Look to the class

The class structure can also yield clues about an upcoming test. Which topics have been singled out for greater emphasis or more detailed explanation? Does the instructor emphasize details or global ideas? Does she refer to the book often, or do her lectures tend to stray from, or greatly enhance, the textbook material?

Some instructors give optional review sessions before an examination. In such a case, attend the session and be prepared. Write down questions you want to ask before the examination. If you have a study guide that accompanies your textbook, use these questions and activities to study. Some test questions may be directly taken from the study guide.

Creating a study plan

Get started early when studying for an upcoming test. Most instructors explain at the beginning of the semester when tests will be administered. Note test dates in your semester calendar. If the dates haven't been announced, ask the instructor for approximate dates of the examinations.

What, where, when?

Create an organized, continuous study plan. Each day, plan how much time you'll devote to studying, what time of day you'll study, and where you'll study. If you plan to study with a partner, set up the meeting times early. Plan enough time to review lecture notes several times and to rehearse the information.

Give yourself at least a week to study for an examination. Studying every day of the week before a test keeps the material fresh and clear in your mind. Reviewing your notes after each class is recommended for helping you understand and keep up with the material but, when preparing for a test, more intense review is also needed.

Pop goes the pop quiz

Sometimes instructors will give an unannounced in-class quiz. In case of a pop quiz, you'll be glad you reviewed material covered in each class.

Let's get together

Gather review materials together. Compile information about the main terms, facts, concepts, themes, problems, questions, and issues stressed in the lectures. The most likely sources for this information include course notes and the textbook.

The textbook's index and glossary are valuable resources for finding important topics and definitions of key terms. Supplementary reading and handouts supplied by the instructor should also be available for review. Keep in mind that material assigned by the instructor—but not discussed in class—may appear on the test in addition to information covered in class.

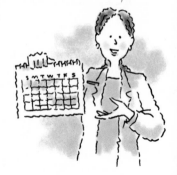

Putting a calendar in the room where you study will help keep you organized, motivated, and on track. Circle the exam date and write down what you'll study each day.

Once is never enough!

When you begin reviewing your class notes in preparation for an examination, make sure to go over your notes and reading materials more than once. Don't expect to remember everything about a topic in one reading.

The first pass at the material serves to refresh your recall of the information and lay a foundation for subsequent passes. Each review becomes easier than the last because the information is fresh and you can anticipate the next topic or sequence of ideas. Take a break between review sessions to let your brain ponder relationships within the material.

Legal cheat sheets

Condense your notes to a one-page summary sheet. Then reconstruct the notes from memory, picturing the placement of notes on the page. Gain command of the material by reciting details. Using these review techniques for various types of tests will help boost your memory:

• For math or science testing, drill yourself by rewriting equations and graphs. Practice writing mathematical symbols so you can reproduce them easily. Practice solving sample problems. If you have particular trouble with certain mathematical expressions or graphs, write them out separately and keep them with you to look at from time to time.

• For short-answer tests, make a list of important terms and write the definition of each. Think of an example for each term.

• For essay questions, look at old essay assignments and examinations. Choose a topic that relates to what you've been learning in class. Write an outline and thesis statement; then flesh out the essay, giving yourself as much time as you would have for a real examination.

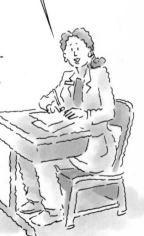

Quiet room, "Do not disturb" sign on my door, cell phone is off, 90 minutes to take the test...I think I'm ready for this practice test!

Dress rehearsal

For every test, try to compile a simulated test based on material from your instructor or review questions in your textbook. Administer the test under testlike conditions, in a quiet room where you will not be disturbed or distracted, allowing yourself the length of time alloted for the actual test. This dress rehearsal will familiarize you with the testing conditions and may alleviate some of your anxiety about facing an unfamiliar situation.

Forming a study group

Many students find that studying in a group setting helps in reviewing and learning class content — especially for difficult subject matters. Teaching is a good way to learn.

Explaining the material to another student not only helps that student, but also gives the person explaining the information an effective way to review the material. A study group is as productive and successful as the group wishes to make it, and following some guidelines will help to ensure its success.

It isn't a party

Use caution when joining or forming a study group. It helps to review the material with others and hear their interpretation of material, but the membership and format of the group need to be conducive to learning. The size of the group is important; four or five members is best. A group that's too big can easily break into smaller groups to discuss different topics and will likely turn into a loud get-together.

Keep your eye on the prize

The members must be committed to learning the material and contributing to discussions to help the group accomplish the task at hand. The members must be compatible and able to put aside differences and concentrate on the work. They must also be reliable and punctual, and be available to attend most of the study meetings.

It helps to assign a time-keeper and a gate-keeper for the study sessions. The time-keeper can alert group members when they need to move on to a different topic. The gate-keeper can help the group stay focused on the subject and keep each meeting from becoming a visiting session.

Come to the group meeting prepared to study and with a basic understanding of the material to be covered. Don't expect the group members to do all the studying for you. Come prepared to explain the material in your own words. If you're having a hard time understanding parts of the material, write down specific questions to ask the group.

Test day

On the day of the test, you can take several actions to make sure you do your best on the examination, including:
- resting
- eating small meals
- avoiding caffeinated drinks and foods
- exercising briefly
- having your test materials ready to go
- getting to class on time, without rushing
- reading the test directions carefully
- budgeting test time efficiently.

Pretest care and feeding

You should get at least 6 hours of sleep the night before a test. In addition, try to wake up at your regular time and eat a normal breakfast without breaking routine. Don't overeat; doing so will cause your body to work harder on digesting the meal than on coming up with correct test answers.

Be careful as well not to overstimulate yourself with caffeinated drinks and foods. Caffeine-related stimulation can distract you and make you jittery for the test.

Brief exercise before a test can invigorate your mind by increasing cerebral circulation. Be careful not to exercise too much, though; exercise just enough to get your blood moving.

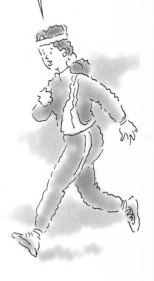

A short, leisurely jog is just what I need to wake up my mind before a test.

Last-minute fact check

Review your summary sheet casually. If you have last-minute facts or formulas to remember, commit them to memory as close to examination time as possible. This information will most likely be stored in short-term memory and won't last long. Jot these facts down as soon as the test begins.

Be prepared

Gather all the supplies you'll need for the examination, especially a watch and extra pencils. During a timed test, you may worry excessively if you don't know how long you've been working and how much time is left. Bring pencils, erasers, paper, a calculator, and other items as needed and allowed.

Make sure to prepare your supplies well in advance of the test so you aren't rushing around immediately before you head to the examination. In fact, you might consider keeping these items in a test kit, which you can grab before each test and restock afterward. The night before a test, put the test kit with your car keys or other items you know you'll be taking to the test, so you won't forget it.

Dress for success

Dress comfortably in layers. If the room is hot, peel off a layer. If it's cold, add a sweater. Bring an easy-to-eat snack and some water if you think you may become distracted by hunger or thirst.

The early bird catches the best seat

Arrive 5 to 10 minutes early for your test. Select the seat you want, preferably one with the least potential for distractions. If the room is poorly lit, sit beneath a light fixture. Stay away from seats near the door. If you still have time, continue reviewing your condensed notes. Avoid listening to other students chat among themselves, especially if they're discussing the examination. Their conversation may make you unduly anxious and needlessly concerned about material you already know well.

Get the 411

When you take your first look at the test, don't let your eye jump to the first question. Instead, read the instructions and listen carefully to verbal instructions. Underline, circle, or otherwise mark important instructions, such as "fill in the circles," "copy the question," or "show your work." Look at the sample questions if there are any, and work them through. (See *Facts and formulas*.)

Next, skim through the test for an overall sense of the questions and their level of difficulty. Read the questions that require lengthy writing. By reviewing the questions in advance, your brain can work on answers to longer questions while you're addressing shorter questions.

In essay questions, underline key words and jot down notes you don't want to forget when you come back to answer the questions completely. For example, you may want to write dates or points you want to make for a question you plan to answer last.

So many questions, so little time

After reading the instructions and previewing the test, determine a budget for your test time. Consider:
- how much time you've been given to complete the examination
- the total number of questions
- the type and difficulty of each question
- the point value for each question.

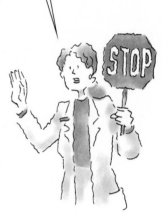

Even if you're eager to start the test, it's important to read the instructions first.

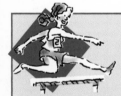

Overcoming obstacles

Facts and formulas

Do you have questions about the best way to remember formulas for a test? If you do, you can probably relate to this student's question—and learn from the answer!

Question
When I get to the calculations on the test, I spend a lot of time trying to remember the correct formulas. This wastes a lot of my time. Any suggestions?

Words of wisdom
When you're in the process of taking a test, you may need to concentrate for a while when trying to remember complicated formulas, facts, conversions, or equations. Prepare to answer such questions before you ever see the first question on the test. Immediately after receiving the test and test instructions, turn your test over and, on the back of the page, write down any conversions, formulas, dates, or facts that you've committed to short-term memory or that you think you may forget. You can then focus on answering the test questions, confident that you can refer back to these notes when necessary.

If you have a choice of questions, decide which ones you intend to answer and in which order you plan to answer them. If, during the test, you start to lag behind the schedule you set, be flexible. Rebound by deciding how you can best use your remaining time.

Types of tests

You may be faced with any combination of test formats, each of which requires its own strategies. Types of tests include:
• objective tests
• subjective tests
• other types of tests (vocabulary, reading comprehension, open-book, take-home, oral, and standardized tests).

Objective tests

In an *objective test*, only one correct answer to a question is possible. These tests primarily measure your ability to recall information. Objective questions are commonly used in standardized examinations. Types of objective tests include:
• multiple-choice
• true-false
• short-answer
• sentence-completion
• problem-solving. (See chapter 9, Preparing for the NCLEX®, for information on NCLEX®-style questions.)

First things first

For all objective tests, start by looking over the entire test to determine the number of questions you'll need to answer. Try to answer the questions in the order they appear. Mark difficult questions, and then move on; you can return to them in the time you have left after you've reached the end of the test. You may be better able to handle these difficult questions at the end of the test, after your brain has had a chance to think about them. In addition, other questions may prompt you to remember the correct answers to the more difficult questions.

Multiple-choice tests

Observe these principles when taking a multiple-choice test:
• Read each question carefully. *Qualifying phrases*, such as *except* and *all of the following*, provide important clues to the correct answer.

- Think of an answer before looking at the options. Then try to match your answer to one of the options. Even if you find a match right away, read all the answers anyway. You may find that another option comes closer to the answer you originally thought correct.
- Use the process of elimination to narrow your choices. Eliminating clearly wrong options greatly improves your odds of selecting the correct answer.
- Work at a good pace. Read each question through, answer it, and then move on to the next question.

Is that your final answer?

Sometimes, test instructions tell you to select the "best" answer. In such a case, there may be more than one correct answer, but one may be better or more appropriate than the others. In these cases, prioritize to determine which response best answers the question.

When prioritizing, think of well-known principles or theories. For example, for a question that asks what you would do first, think of Maslow's hierarchy of needs. Physical needs are always more important than psychological needs, so meeting nutritional demands would automatically come before establishing a trusting relationship.

Anything's possible

In a well-constructed test, all options are plausible. Therefore, go back to the question and look for a clue that makes one answer better than the others (such as the word *first* in the question: "What should the nurse do first?").

Don't be rash

Some test makers deliberately put a plausible — but incorrect — answer first. To avoid simply picking the first answer that appears, read all answers before deciding which is correct.

When it's right, it's right

Sometimes, questions and correct responses are taken directly out of the textbook, review guides, computer programs, or lecture notes. If you recognize particular words or phrases in one of the options, or if the question and one option seem like the right combination, choose that option; it's probably the correct one.

Be alert for "attractive distracters," words that *look like* the word to be defined but aren't. For example, if *illusion* is the correct answer, *allusion* might be used as a "decoy" among the answers.

The homestretch

When you've finished the test:

> **Memory jogger**
>
> **REAP** your rewards of great grades when taking multiple-choice tests! Remember these steps:
>
> **R**ead each question carefully.
>
> **E**liminate wrong answers.
>
> **A**ttempt to match your answer with an option.
>
> **P**ace yourself.

> Some tests offer more than one correct response. Read all of the responses and choose the best answer.

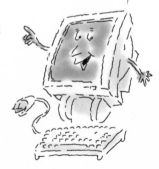

• go back and read the instructions again to make sure you've followed them
• check that you've answered the questions in the areas where they were supposed to be answered
• check the questions you flagged for further review
• review all the questions if you have time.

Change answers only if you're convinced they need to be changed to be correct. Trust your first impressions; they're usually accurate.

True-false tests

In general, *true-false questions* assess your recognition of information rather than your ability to recall it and concentrate on simple facts and details. Most true-false statements are straightforward and are based on key words or phrases from the textbook or lectures. Always decide whether the statement is completely true before you mark it true. If only part of it is true, then the whole statement is false.

Take the hint

One word can turn an otherwise true statement into a false one, or a false statement into a true one. Pay special attention to these words:
• all
• always
• because
• generally
• never
• none
• only
• sometimes
• usually.

> Be on the lookout for small words, such as *always* and *never*. They're valuable clues in your search for the correct response.

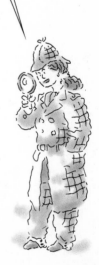

Short-answer and sentence-completion tests

Short-answer test items usually consist of one or two specific sentences after which you're asked to give a definition or formula. *Sentence-completion items* typically consist of a single sentence in which you're asked to fill in a specific word or phrase.

Plan of attack

To take a short-answer or sentence-completion test, break the items into these three categories:

Items you know without hesitation

Questions you should be able to answer if you think for a minute

Items about which you have no idea.

Answer the questions you know first. Then attack the questions that need more thought. Lastly, answer all remaining questions as best you can.

Don't blank out on blanks

Sentence-completion, or *fill-in-the-blank*, questions generally ask for an exact wording from memory. Make sure the grammar is consistent. When in doubt, guess; even if you make a generalized guess, you may receive partial credit. Many times, the question itself will contain a clue to the correct answer. For example, a date may help you narrow the scope of answers simply by providing a point of historical reference.

The numbers game

Look at the number and length of blanks in the question, and use them as clues to the correct answer. Is there more than one blank? Are the blanks long or short? Many instructors deliberately indicate when they expect one word, two words, or three words by using that number of blanks. The instructor may also use long blanks for long answers and short blanks for short answers.

Problem-solving tests

Tests that require problem-solving skills are used mainly in quantitative subjects, such as math and science. To approach a problem-solving examination, first read through all of the problems before answering them. Underline key words in the instructions and important data in the problems. Jot down thoughts that come to mind, such as specific formulas or possible approaches to solving the problems. As you move from question to question, repeat the same procedure.

Easy does it

Work on the easiest problems first; return to the more difficult ones later. Working on simple problems first will help build your confidence and warm up your brain for the more difficult problems to come.

Nothing to hide

Show all of your work. If you make a mistake, the instructor can see where you went wrong and may at least give you partial credit. Be careful and deliberate about your calculations so you don't make computational errors. Check that your answer meets all of the requirements of the problem. In addition, check that your answer makes sense. If your answer indicates that you would give a patient 20 pills, does that make sense? If not, check your work again.

If at first you don't succeed...

If you have trouble solving a problem, approach it in a different manner. Think about similar problems from class or homework and the methods used to solve them. These are typically the methods used in the test, except that the ones in the test use different numbers or scenarios. Keep in mind that there's usually more than one way to solve a problem. If one method doesn't work, try another.

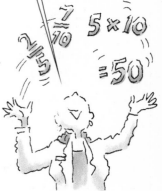

Partial credit is better than none at all! Show all your calculations and your instructor may give you a break — even if your answer isn't correct.

Subjective tests

In a *subjective test*, such as an essay test, no single correct answer exists. Instead, the person grading the test judges how well each essay demonstrates understanding of the material. Follow these steps for successfully completing an essay test:

✋ Read all instructions, underlining important words and phrases.

✌ Read all questions even if you need to answer only some of them. Jot down facts and thoughts about each topic.

🤟 Mark the time you estimate it will take to complete each question.

🖖 Outline your answer.

🖐 Write the answer.

🖐 ✌ Read the instructions and question again. Review your answer. Proofread, and make corrections.

Stop and get directions

Read all instructions first. Failure to do so can result in points being deducted. For instance, the instructions may state to supply three supporting facts for each point of view. If you provide only one or two facts, you may lose points.

When reading the instructions for the first time, underline key points so you can refer to them quickly as you write. Unless the instructions state otherwise, double-space your essay and write only on the right-hand pages of the test booklet. Both techniques provide room for information to be added and for comments from the instructor.

Take it from me! Reading the instructions first will ensure that you take your test correctly. (Afterward, you can come help me with this bicycle!)

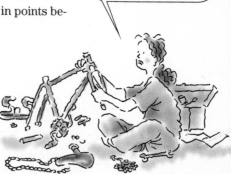

Advice from the experts

Five-paragraph format

The *five-paragraph format* is an easy-to-follow structure for answering an essay question that asks you to state and support an opinion. Use it to get yourself started, especially when pressed for time.

Paragraph	Content
1	Introduction, in which you briefly outline the direction your argument will take and list the three main points you'll illustrate
2	First point, including at least two supporting facts
3	Second point, including at least two supporting facts
4	Third point, including at least two supporting facts
5	Conclusion, which pulls together the three main points into one final summary statement

Leave no question unread

After reading all instructions, read all the questions, quickly jotting down what you know about each topic, including facts, formulas, names, dates, ideas, and impressions. Later, when you write your outline, you'll have facts and figures handy to plug into the essay quickly. In addition, if you have a choice of questions for the test, you'll know which topics you know the most about by looking at how many notes you've written for each.

Time is money — and 90% of your grade

If a single essay question is worth, say, 50% of your grade, plan to spend 50% of your time on that question. Break this time allotment down further to include the time required to organize an outline, write the essay, and check your work.

Birth of an outline

When creating an outline, first write your thesis statement to guide you in writing the rest of the essay. Choose a title, even if one isn't required. The title, like the thesis, helps guide the direction of your arguments.

When organizing your outline, use the five-paragraph format as a guide. (See *Five-paragraph format*.) Content and organization

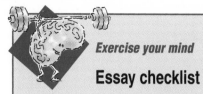

Exercise your mind

Essay checklist

After completing an essay question, check your work. Ask yourself these questions to determine whether you've covered all the points you intended to cover.

Content

• Did you stick to your original point of view?

• Have you proven each argument?

• Have you provided examples?

• Have you clearly distinguished facts from opinions?

• Have you mentioned exceptions to your general statements?

Organization

• Did you open with a topic sentence?

• Does the topic sentence address the question?

• Did you follow your outline?

• Did you cover all the points in your original outline?

• Does your ending pull together all points without adding new information?

Writing mechanics

• Does every sentence state what you intended it to state?

• Are you sure of the meanings of all the words?

• Are spelling, grammar, punctuation, and sentence structure correct?

• Is your work neat and your handwriting legible?

typically account for most of your test grade. If you run out of time while writing an essay, you may be able to submit your outline, which shows your organization and intent.

Get to the point

Follow your outline when you write, and get to the point quickly. Your thesis statement should restate the question or answer the question succinctly. Use the introduction to tell the instructor what you're going to say. If the question states to "explain" or "summarize," for example, be sure to do just that. (See *Essay checklist.*)

Guided by your outline, make your points and supporting statements in the body of the essay. Each paragraph should have a

Advice from the experts

Writing mechanics for essay questions

Answering an essay question involves providing the correct information, of course, but it also involves presenting the information in a readable format. Like a finely tuned car, a finely crafted essay shows that the author pays attention to mechanical details. Following certain tips for mechanically precise writing will help you write clear, compelling answers to essay questions.

Punctuation and word choice

• Avoid semicolons, exclamation marks, and parenthetical statements. Many inexperienced writers use semicolons incorrectly and exclamation marks too frequently. Parenthetical statements can knock a sentence off track.

• Avoid using a big word when a smaller one will do. Using unnecessarily long words or jargon can confuse your reader and detract from the clarity of your response. Keep it simple, and your instructor will be able to judge your knowledge more clearly.

• Avoid fragments and run-ons. A *fragment* is an incomplete sentence, such as *Because the laboratory technologist is responsible for monitoring blood bank supplies.* A *run-on* is a long sentence typically formed by joining two or three other sentences without using proper punctuation or linking words.

• Avoid slang, nonstandard language, and profanity. Keep your tone professional throughout.

Content and transitions

• Support all opinions with facts or other supporting information.

• Use transitions properly to give your writing a smooth flow. For example, if you introduce a term or concept at the end of one paragraph, use the term or refer to the concept in the first sentence of the next paragraph.

• When working on lined paper, skip every other line as you write. Skipping lines makes it easier for the instructor to read your response and also allows for extra room in which to write additional information later.

topic statement, which, in turn, should relate to your thesis statement. Incorporate the facts and thoughts you jotted down at the beginning of the test. Write simple, direct, specific sentences that follow one another logically.

The conclusion should restate your thesis, drawing together the points made in the body of the essay. The conclusion tells the instructor that you had a point to make and that you made it.

Nips and tucks

When you've finished writing your essay, go back and read the question and instructions again. Make sure you've answered the question and that you've addressed all the points in the instructions. Then read your essay slowly and carefully, proofreading for grammatical errors and legibility. (See *Writing mechanics for essay questions.*) Make corrections where necessary.

Know when to fold 'em

After you've reviewed your completed essay and you've corrected errors and made needed changes, stop writing! Additional, extraneous verbiage will be viewed by your instructor as just that. When the question has been answered as it was intended to be, any other additions or changes are more likely to hurt your grade than to help. They'll also obscure the main points your instructor will be looking for.

Other types of tests

Other types of tests include:
• vocabulary
• reading comprehension
• open-book and take-home
• oral
• standardized.

Vocabulary tests

A *vocabulary test* assesses your ability to remember the meaning of a word or use it correctly. Vocabulary tests are commonly used when studying foreign languages or in fields that employ specialized terminology.

Winning with words

These strategies are useful when you're faced with a vocabulary test:
• Avoid decoy options that look like the correct answer but aren't.
• Choose grammatically correct answers only.
• If you don't know the meaning of a word, try to remember where you've heard it and how it was used in a sentence. Select the answer that seems closest in meaning.
• Try to determine what part of speech the word is — for example, is it a noun or verb? Knowing a word's part of speech helps put the word into grammatical context and give you a clue about the meaning.
• Apply your knowledge of other languages. If you studied Latin, for instance, you may be able to derive the correct answer by looking at the unknown word's root. Look also at the word's prefix or suffix for clues.

Reading comprehension tests

In a *reading comprehension test*, you'll be asked to read a particular passage and then answer questions based on the passage. For these tests, read the *questions* first and then the passage. That way, you can focus on finding answers to the questions as you read.

Just the facts, Ma'am

After you read the passage, base your answers entirely on facts given in the passage. Applying outside knowledge can cost you points. Check your answers to make sure you've answered the questions completely.

Open-book and take-home tests

In an *open-book* or *take-home examination*, you're allowed to refer to your textbooks or notes. These tests deemphasize memorization and encourage critical thinking. They're often graded more strictly than tests based on your ability to eliminate factual errors. Neatness and grammar may count more heavily because you're given time to find and correct those errors.

Getting to know all about you

Here are some strategies for taking an open-book or take-home examination:
- Use the index and table of contents extensively.
- Don't copy your essays from the book. Use as many sources and resources as you're allowed. Treat the assignment like writing a paper.
- For some open-book tests, the instructor may allow students to bring only one page of notes. In such a case, organize and condense as much information as possible onto that one paper.
- Check your answers. Make sure you answered the questions without adding new, unsupported thoughts at the end.
- Proofread your work.

Oral examinations

In an oral examination, you need to speak clearly, fluently, and without much time to prepare an answer. If you're allowed to choose a topic in advance, prepare as completely as if you were writing an essay. Choose a relatively narrow topic on which you can remain focused and for which you can give many supporting details. Try to make at least three points during the examination, and support each point with three pieces of evidence.

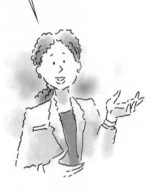

If you glance at the questions first in a reading comprehension test, then you can look for answers while you read the passage.

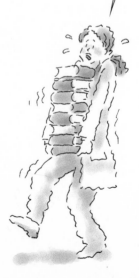

Open-book tests have their advantages — especially if you happen to own a forklift!

Say it again, Sam

Practice for an oral examination the same way you would prepare for a written test. Rehearse your answers in a simulated testing situation. Practice public speaking so you feel comfortable speaking in front of an audience.

Here are some tips to help you get through your oral examinations:

• Dress appropriately and look neat. Your physical appearance can make a positive or negative impression on your audience.

• Maintain control of your voice. Speak clearly and in measured tones. Avoid speaking quickly, mumbling, or letting your voice become too excited and "squeaky."

• Look at your audience. If you can't look directly at someone in the audience, look at a reference point in the audience. Looking at a reference point gives audience members the impression that you're looking at them. You might also look just above the heads of the people in the audience.

• If the oral examination involves giving a speech, prepare notes and do most of your speaking without reading. If you read directly from your notes, you might sound ill-prepared.

• Use language you're comfortable with. Don't use offensive language or words you don't know how to pronounce. In preparing, practice pronouncing the names of people or places that may come up during your test.

• Treat questions seriously. If you're allowed to take notes, write down questions asked of you. This is particularly helpful if the question contains several parts. If you don't understand what the questioner is asking, request clarification. Always repeat or rephrase the question yourself so you're sure you understand it.

• Unless you know how to answer a question immediately, take a moment to organize your thoughts before you begin your response.

• If you don't know the answer to a question, explain why. Perhaps the answer falls outside your realm of expertise.

• Exit gracefully. When your oral examination is finished, collect yourself and your papers and thank the audience members for their attention.

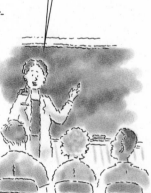

How am I speaking? Practice will help me speak clearly and fluently during my oral examination.

Standardized tests

Standardized tests — for example, the Graduate Record Examination (GRE), Millers Analogy Test (MAT), and Scholastic Aptitude Test (SAT) — are used for placement and admissions pur-poses. The test scores for standardized tests become a permanent part of your academic record.

Always prepare before taking a standardized test by practicing under simulated test conditions. Use materials prepared by the same people who publish the actual test or materials designed specifically to replicate the actual test.

Numerous practice books and software are available for nearly every major standardized test. Take advantage of these books, using their self-tests to practice under simulated test conditions. Practice questions may also be available on the Internet, depending on the test.

Test review

Tests provide you and your instructor with valuable information to evaluate your performance and judge your progress. Most instructors review the tests with the class after the examination. Review your examination when it's returned to you. (See *Test review checklist.*) Reflect carefully on instructor comments on the test, especially comments on an essay test. They can tell you not only about mistakes you've made but also how you can better fulfill that particular instructor's expectations and better perform on the final examination.

Exercise your mind

Test review checklist

Reviewing your test after it has been corrected can help clarify where you went wrong and what areas you need to concentrate on for the next test. After your test is returned to you, ask yourself these questions:

• What was my biggest problem overall?

• In general, what types of comments did the instructor make?

• Did I prepare for this test properly?

• Did I make careless errors? If so, how can I avoid doing the same in the future?

• What else can I learn from my mistakes?

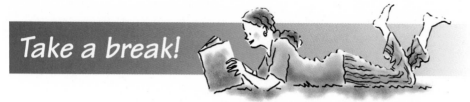

Take a break!

Scrambled or over-easy

Do you experience anxiety before a test? Fill in the blanks and then unscramble the circled letters to reveal a technique you can use to cope with your anxiety. Find the answers on the next page.

1. This is the best antidote for test anxiety.

— — —◯— — — — —

2. This is the minimum number of hours of sleep advised the night before a test.

—◯—

3. Avoid consuming this before a test to prevent jitteriness.

— — — —◯— — —

4. This type of test has only one correct answer per question.

◯— — — — — — — —

5. No single correct answer exists when taking this type of test.

— — — — — — —◯— —

6. Creating one of these will help you organize your thoughts to answer a question.

— —◯— — — —

7. This pulls together the three main points of an essay.

— — — — — — — — —◯

8. This is the first thing you should read when you get a test.

— — — — — — —◯— — —

9. This type of test assesses your ability to remember the meaning of a word.

— — —◯— — — —

10. Problem-solving skills are commonly used for testing in this subject.

◯— — —

Answer: _____

Answer key

S T U (D) Y I N G

S (I) X

C A F F (E) I N E

(O) B J E C T I V E

S U B J E C T (I) V E

O U (T) L I N E

C O N C L U S I O (N)

I N S T R U C (T) I O N S

V O C (A) B U L A R Y

(M) A T H

You can use MEDITATION to cope with your anxiety before a test.

Stress? What stress?

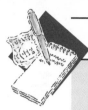

Just the facts

In this chapter, you'll learn:

♦ how stress is the body's response to a demand

♦ how the body responds to stress

♦ how stress management techniques can be directed at the body or the mind.

What is stress?

Stress, according to the famed neuropsychologist Hans Selye, is "the nonspecific response of the body to any demands made upon it." When faced with a stimulus, the body seeks to adapt. These adaptations provoke a variety of physical and psychological reactions that, collectively, we recognize as stress.

People typically think of stress as being negative or unpleasant, but that isn't always the case. The way we react to stress will, in large part, determine the type of impact stress will have on our lives. We can react to stress positively or negatively, depending on the type of stress and our ability to manage it.

Eureka! Eustress!

People commonly encounter situations that cause them to react in a positive way. This response to beneficial environmental stimuli, called *eustress*, helps keep us alert, motivates us to face challenges, and drives us to solve problems. These low levels of stress are manageable and may be thought of as necessary and normal stimulation.

Stop the insanity!

Distress, on the other hand, results when our bodies overreact to events. Distress leads to what has been called the *fight-or-flight response*, a reaction deeply

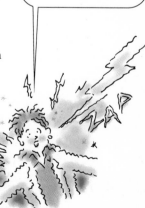

Is this a good look for me? I guess it's just my body's way of adapting to a stressful stimulus.

rooted in human physiology and behavior. The fight-or-flight response evolved as a mechanism to deal with life-or-death situations faced by primitive humans.

Lions, and tigers, and bears — oh my!

Nowadays, truly life-or-death situations tend to occur rarely for most people. Yet the human body continues to react to day-to-day situations the way our ancestors did, as if our lives depended on our reactions. For instance, your body can't physiologically differentiate between the threat of a saber-toothed tiger and that of a boss in a gray tweed suit. How we perceive and interpret the events of life dictates how our body reacts. If we think something is scary or worrisome, our bodies react accordingly.

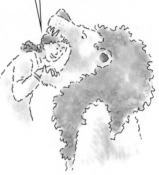

Since primitive times, people have been dealing with stress. Most of us don't have to worry about threatening animals today, though!

Rating your reaction

Exposing two people to the same stressor can provoke very different reactions. One possible explanation for these differences is that people have varying levels of what psychologists call *coherence*, or a sense of fitting into the environment. People with a strong sense of coherence feel more in control of themselves and react more positively to stress than do people with a weaker sense of coherence. Understanding how you tend to react to stress can help you gain control of your reactions and cope with stress more effectively.

Reacting to stress

Selye categorized the body's reactions to environmental stress in three phases, together called the *general adaptation syndrome (GAS)*. The phases of GAS are:

  alarm

  resistance

  exhaustion.

All hands on deck!

In the first stage, *alarm*, a nonspecific, general alarm occurs. In this response, the hypothalamus in the brain activates the autonomic nervous system, which, in turn, sparks activity in the pituitary gland and leads to an arousal of body defenses. At this point, the person experiences an increase in alertness and anxiety.

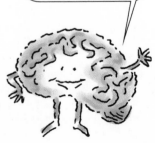

Stress alerts my hypothalamus, which activates the autonomic nervous system and sets body defenses in motion.

Call in the hormones

During the second phase of the GAS, *resistance*, the hormone epinephrine is released from the adrenal glands. Epinephrine helps the body counteract the stressor directly or take flight to avoid the stressor's harmful effects.

Stress overload

If exposure to the same stressor continues over a long period, the body will no longer be able to adapt to or resist the stressor's effects, and *exhaustion* sets in. Regardless of the inner strength of an individual, prolonged, unrelenting stress eventually breaks down the body's resistance, and disease, or even death, can result.

Recognizing stress

Signs and symptoms of stress vary, depending on whether the stress reaction is of short duration or prolonged. Stress can also cause a number of psychological effects.

Stress, I know you all too well

Short-term signs and symptoms of stress are easy to recognize and differ little from person to person. When a person is faced with stress, her:
- breathing becomes rapid and shallow
- heart rate increases
- muscles in the shoulders, forehead, and back of the neck tighten
- hands and feet become cold and sweaty.

Stress can also lead to disturbances in the GI system, such as a "butterfly" stomach or diarrhea, vomiting, and frequent urination. The mouth may become parched, and the hands and knees may begin to shake or tremble. These short-term effects disappear soon after the stressor is removed.

Enough is enough!

Extended exposure to stress can have lasting or even permanent effects on the body. Chronic stress suppresses the immune system by destroying white blood cells (WBCs) and suppressing WBC production, thus diminishing the body's disease-fighting capabilities. In addition, stress causes the release of free fatty acids into the bloodstream. These fatty acids can eventually accumulate as fatty deposits on arterial walls and lead to coronary artery disease, stroke, or heart attack.

Matters of the mind

A number of psychological changes also occur because of stress. Memory becomes blocked, and clear thinking becomes difficult. A stressed individual may also find it difficult to solve problems efficiently. If the situation persists, the person finds it difficult to concentrate and may experience a general sense of fear or anxiety, insomnia, early waking, changes in eating habits, excessive worrying, fatigue, or a frequent urge to escape from the stressor.

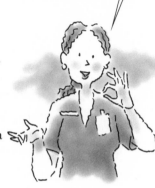

A small amount of stress helps me focus. The key word here is small.

Characteristics of anxious students

Stress from classroom and test situations commonly results in anxiety. (See *Coping with test-taking anxiety.*) Study-related anxiety can affect your performance as a student in several ways. Anxiety appears to improve performance on simple tasks and heavily practiced skills, but it interferes with accomplishment of more complex tasks or skills that aren't thoroughly practiced.

If simple, practiced skills have become boring or rote, a small amount of anxiety can help keep you alert and eager to finish. If a task is difficult or new, however, anxiety can prove distracting, making it more difficult to complete the task successfully.

Advice from the experts

Coping with test-taking anxiety

A test may cause undue anxiety. If you're experiencing worry and anxiety before a test, you can use a number of techniques to help you cope more effectively with your anxiety.

Before the test
• Discuss test content with your instructor and classmates.
• Develop effective study and test preparation skills.
• Spread your final studying over several days rather than cramming right before the test.
• Review your textbook, notes, and homework problems.
• Jot specific concepts or formulas on 3" × 5" cards and then study the cards.
• Take a practice test under examlike conditions.
• Continue your regular exercise program.
• Get sufficient rest the night before the test.

• Emphasize positive aspects of the test when you find yourself thinking negatively.
• Avoid studying immediately before the test.
• Relax or do something non-test-related immediately before the test.
• Arrive at the testing room about 5 minutes early to relax before the test is distributed. Arriving earlier may cause undue anxiety.

During the test
• Do something to break the test atmosphere, if allowed, such as getting a drink, sharpening a pencil, eating a snack, or asking a question.
• Alternately tense and relax muscles in several parts of your body, and then take several deep breaths with your eyes closed.
• Practice calming yourself by saying something like, "I have much more in my life than this test. I am calm and relaxed."
• Visualize a calm, soothing scene whenever you feel anxious.

A stress-filled brain

Highly anxious students seem to divide their attention between the new material and a preoccupation with how nervous they're feeling. So instead of concentrating on a lecture or on what she's reading, an anxious student keeps noticing the tight feelings in her chest, thinking something like, "I'm so tense; I'll never understand this stuff!" Because much of an anxious student's attention is occupied with negative thoughts about performing poorly, being criticized, or feeling embarrassed, she may miss information to be learned.

Distracting distractions

Anxious students tend to have poor study habits. They commonly have trouble learning material if it's somewhat disorganized or difficult to understand, or if it requires them to rely on their memory. Anxious students may be more easily distracted by irrelevant or incidental aspects of the task at hand. They seem to have trouble focusing on significant details and, as a result, waste time.

The deep freeze and forget

Anxious students often know more than they can demonstrate on a test, but because they commonly lack effective test-taking skills, they fail to demonstrate their knowledge when it really counts. They "freeze and forget" in a testing environment even though they may excel in nontest environments. (See *Recognizing the "freeze-up."*)

> This freeze-and-forget stuff can leave you cold! Careful preparation will help warm you up — and a nice, hot bubble bath wouldn't hurt either!

Advice from the experts

Recognizing the "freeze-up"

The most common symptom of test anxiety is experiencing a mental block or "freeze-up." A person with test anxiety may read the test questions and find the words meaningless. Or, the person may need to read test questions several times to fully comprehend them. Other symptoms include:
• feeling panic about not knowing the answer to a question or as time is running out of the test period
• worrying how your performance compares to the performance of other students
• feeling easily distracted during the examination
• plotting ways to escape from a test, such as sneaking out or faking an illness.

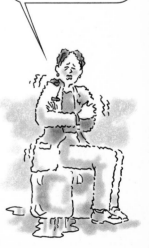

Managing stress

Stress management is a technique that can be useful on many levels. It can be as simple as taking a 5-minute break from studying and as comprehensive as reconsidering your life goals. To truly adjust your reaction to stress, choose the kinds of stress management techniques that will work for you. These techniques include:

- setting priorities
- caring for your body
- caring for your mind
- using social supports.

Setting priorities

A key factor in stress management involves managing the limited amount of time you have. As a student, the activities and responsibilities you need to fit into each day may include going to classes, studying and preparing for class, working, participating in extramural activities, fulfilling family responsibilities, maintaining friendships and other personal relationships, engaging in your favorite hobbies, exercising, and attending social affairs.

Feeling the burden of fitting all those activities into a limited time is a source of significant stress. Setting priorities can help you manage activities and reduce the stress they cause.

The simple life

It seems that we're always faced with more to do than can be accomplished. At times you may feel overwhelmed with responsibility, overextended, and out of control. The answer to a life that seems overwhelming is simplification. As Elaine St. James, a leader of the simplicity movement, states in her book *Simplify Your Life*, "Wise men and women in every major culture throughout history have found that the secret to happiness isn't in getting more but in wanting less." She encourages everyone to take some time out, examine their lives, and set some reasonable and specific goals that will simplify life.

Simplifying your life means identifying what you most want to have and most want to accomplish. Then determine how to reach those goals as simply as possible. For example, you may want to buy an expensive new car. Do you also want the high insurance rates that come with it? Are you ready for the added drain on your finances? Or would you prefer at this point to buy a solid, dependable secondhand car?

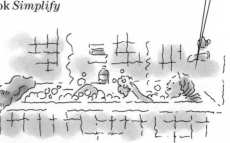

Taking some time for yourself will help you relax, examine your life, and set priorities.

Here are some other ways to simplify your life:

• Run your errands all in one place. Don't hop from one shopping center to another; that takes time and energy. You might have to pay a little more for some of the things you need, but it will be worth it by making one stop instead of five or six.

• Turn off the television.

• Don't answer the phone every time it rings. If you have an answering machine, let it pick up sometimes. Give yourself a break.

• Stop sending greeting cards at Christmas and other holidays.

• Resign from organizations whose meetings you hate to attend.

• Say no to one request each day or week.

• Every once in a while, just do nothing.

Remember, life isn't a race. Take it at your own pace, and simplify.

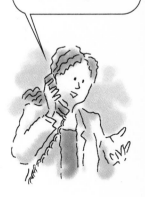

Thank you for your call. At the sound of the tone, please leave a message...

Those drop-dead deadlines

If you can't reduce the number of demands you have, try to increase the time you allow yourself to perform them. Many deadlines are self-imposed. If you're overscheduled in your classes and, as a result, overwhelmed with responsibilities, perhaps you can aim to graduate a semester later. Sometimes it's necessary to differentiate between deadlines that can't be changed and those that can be extended without compromising goals.

Undo the urgency

It's easy to mistake an urgency for an emergency. When you're feeling overwhelmed, sit down and divide a sheet of paper into three columns. Label the columns *Emergency*, *Urgent*, and *Non-urgent*. Then prioritize all the tasks on your to-do list according to whether they're true emergencies (things that *must* be done immediately), urgencies (things that are important but aren't emergencies), or non-urgent. A bathtub that's leaking water through the ceiling into the kitchen is an emergency; handle it right away. If the tub is partly plugged but still drains and isn't leaking, it's urgent; handle it as soon as you have time. A bathtub that works fine but needs to be cleaned is non-urgent; handle it the next time you clean the bathroom.

Tasks that don't fit into any of the columns aren't important. Take them off your list, or put them on a separate list titled *Things to do sometime, maybe*. Above all, keep other people's needs in mind but don't sacrifice your needs and your health for things that aren't emergencies or urgencies.

Arranging the sock drawer

Organize your schedule to make the most of what time is available. Identify and reduce wasted time, delegating certain activities to others in your social network and avoiding taking on too much yourself. Eliminate tasks if they aren't a high priority. That way you can schedule more time for high-priority tasks.

Nobody's perfect!

Another problem that affects optimal use of time is striving for perfection with each task, thereby delaying the task's completion. Give yourself permission to be imperfect. Not every task requires perfect effort. That doesn't mean you should do sloppy work, but it does mean you should avoid laboring over tasks until the outcome is what you consider perfect.

Delegate household tasks and chores to roommates or family members, such as your spouse or children. Don't expect perfection or that the task will be accomplished exactly as you would do it. Allow for imperfections, and be glad that someone else is taking care of things. This can also help your friends and family feel that they're helping you achieve your goals.

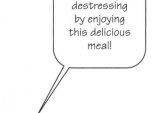

I'm destressing by enjoying this delicious meal!

Baby steps

Be aware of procrastination that stems from feeling unable to complete a task. If a task seems overwhelming, break it down into smaller tasks that can be done individually. It's better to start with a small step than not to start at all.

Caring for your body

Because stress prompts a physical response from the body, caring for your body properly plays an important role in your ability to manage stress effectively. Caring for your body involves exercising, getting sufficient rest, eating well, and engaging in stress-reducing breathing activities.

Exercise

Many students complain about not having enough time to study, let alone exercise. However, finding the time to exercise — even if it's just a daily regimen of stretches in the morning — can help lower stress, keep you looking and feeling trim, and make you feel better all around. Rather than draining energy, regular exercise actually replenishes your energy supply, allowing you to more easily manage all of the tasks you need to complete each day. Knowing what kinds of activities are best and how long and how often to exercise is the first step on the path to a healthy body.

Use it or lose it

Aerobic activities, such as swimming, jogging, brisk walking, cycling, or engaging in a vigorous racquet sport, not only strengthen your cardiovascular system but also provide numerous other physiologic benefits. For instance, people who engage in aerobic exercise tend to have more energy, feel less stress, sleep better, lose weight more easily, and experience an improved self-image.

The buddy system

In choosing your type of exercise, select an activity you enjoy. Unless you enjoy it, you won't continue with it. You might also look for an exercise partner to provide companionship, camaraderie, and motivation to exercise on a regular basis.

Take a day off

Exercise at least three times per week for at least 20 to 30 minutes at a time. You'll see even greater improvements if you build gradually to four to six times weekly. Give yourself at least one day per week free of exercise so your body can rest properly.

Rest

People experiencing high levels of stress tend to get insufficient amounts of sleep and become fatigued. Fatigue by itself is a stressor, which increases the amount of stress you feel, which leads to more fatigue, and so on. Sometimes it's more important to get some rest than to complete every task on your daily to-do list. Listen to your body when it tells you it's tired. After all, your body knows best when it's time to rest!

> When your body says it's time to sleep, it's nap time!

Eating right

A balanced, nutritious diet is essential for maintaining good health. Diet also may influence your ability to cope with stress. Studies have shown that eating an adequate breakfast each day can improve the body's reaction to stress. Hunger can make an individual less able to cope effectively with stress.

An apple a day

During periods of stress, increase your intake of fruits and vegetables to supply vitamins B and C and folic acid, all of which enhance your body's ability to deal with the stress. Foods that can help elevate your mood include those that contain the amino acid tryptophan, such as milk, eggs, poultry, legumes, nuts, and cereal.

Got milk?

Reducing your consumption of coffee, tea, cola soft drinks, and drugs containing caffeine can help control stress. Caffeine stimulates the sympathetic nervous system and promotes tension and anxiety. Avoid high-glucose foods as well; they can lead to sudden increases and decreases in blood glucose, which affect your ability to concentrate.

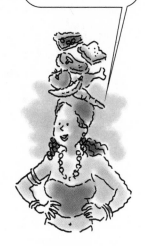

Fruits and vegetables are some of the best stressbusters. They work much better when you eat them than when you wear them!

Stress-reduction techniques

A number of stress-reduction techniques — including conscious relaxation, massage, relaxation breathing, yoga, and other meditation-based activities — can be used to counteract your body's damaging reactions to stress.

Unwind those muscles

Relaxation is a conscious attempt to relax your muscles. Because tension tends to target muscles in the head, neck, and shoulders, many relaxation techniques focus on those parts of the body.

Here's an example of one relaxation technique. Relax your neck and shoulders. Slowly drop your head forward, roll it gently to the center of your right shoulder, and pause. Gently roll it to the center of your left shoulder, and pause. Roll it gently forward to the center of your chest, and pause. Reverse direction and go from left to right. Your goal for this and other forms of conscious relaxation is to slowly stretch muscles into relaxation. Similar techniques can be used to relax your entire body. (See *Full-body relaxation*.)

Therapeutic massage

Therapeutic massage today is used primarily for stress reduction and relaxation. The primary physiologic effect of therapeutic massage is improved blood circulation and muscle relaxation. As the muscles are kneaded and stretched, blood return to the heart increases and toxins such as lactic acid are carried out of the muscle tissue to be excreted from the body.

Enter endorphins

Improved circulation also results in increased perfusion and oxygenation of tissues. Improved oxygenation of the brain helps us think more clearly and, psychologically, helps us to feel relaxed and more alive. Massage also appears to trigger the release of endorphins, the body's natural pain relievers.

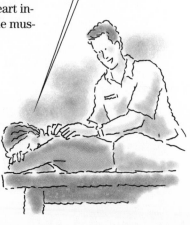

Massage triggers endorphins, which help relieve pain. Now that's what I call therapy!

Advice from the experts

Full-body relaxation

Relaxation exercises not only reduce stress but also send more blood and oxygen to the muscles. As muscles relax, they stretch, which allows more blood to flow into them. As a result, they gradually feel warmer and heavier. To relax your entire body in an attempt to reduce stress, try this exercise.

Start at the feet
Begin by settling back into a comfortable position. Start by focusing on relaxing your feet and ankles. Wiggle your feet or toes to help them to relax, and then allow that wave of relaxation to continue into the muscles of the calves. Continue the process up to the muscles of the thighs. Your legs should gradually feel more and more comfortable and relaxed.

Upper body
Next, concentrate on relaxing the muscles of your spine. Feel the relaxation spread into your abdomen. As you do this, you might feel a pleasant sense of warmth spreading to other parts of your body.

Focus on the muscles of the chest. Each time you exhale, your chest muscles should relax a little more. Let this relaxation flow into the muscles of the shoulders and then the arms and hands. Gradually, your arms and hands will become heavy, limp, and warm.

Neck and head
Now concentrate on relaxing the muscles of the neck, imagining that the muscles are as floppy as a handful of rubber bands. Next, relax the muscles of the jaws, cheeks, and sides of the face. Relax the eyes, nose, forehead, and scalp.

Cleansing breath
Lastly, take a long, slow, deep breath to eliminate tension that may remain.

Qigong
Qigong (pronounced "chee goong") is a system of gentle exercise, meditation, and controlled breathing used by millions of Chinese people daily to increase strength and relax the mind. Practitioners believe that when practiced daily over time, *qigong* can improve strength and flexibility, reverse damage due to injury or disease, relieve pain, restore energy, and induce relaxation and healing.

Yoga
One of the oldest known health practices, *yoga* (which means *union* in Sanskrit) is the integration of physical, mental, and spiritual energies to promote health and wellness. The basic components of yoga include proper breathing, movement, and posture. While practicing specific postures, the practitioner pays close attention to his breathing, exhaling at certain times and inhaling at others. The breathing techniques are believed to promote relaxation and enhance the vital flow of energy known as *prana*.

Controlled breathing with gentle exercise and meditation can help you relax and reduce stress.

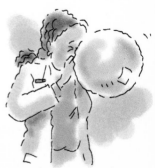

Numerous scientific studies have shown that the regular practice of yoga can produce the same physiologic changes as meditation. Known as the *relaxation response*, these changes include decreased heart and respiratory rates, improved cardiac and respiratory function, decreased blood pressure, decreased oxygen consumption, increased alpha wave activity, and EEG synchronicity, a change in brain wave activity that occurs only in deep meditation.

Tai chi chuan

A form of exercise built on the mind-body connection, *tai chi chuan* (or *tai chi*) combines physical movement, meditation, and breathing to induce relaxation and improve balance, posture, co-ordination, endurance, strength, and flexibility. Tai chi also benefits patients who suffer from anxiety, stress, restlessness, and depression. Tai chi can be practiced by people of all ages, sizes, and physical abilities because it relies more on technique than on strength. Participants perform a series of rhythmic movement patterns slowly and methodically.

Imagery

In *imagery*, imagination is used to promote relaxation, relieve symptoms (or help to better cope with them), and heal disease. Imagery is based on the principle that the mind and body are interconnected and can work together to encourage healing. Imagery can lower blood pressure and decrease heart rate. It can also affect brain wave activity, oxygen supply to the tissues, vascular constriction, skin temperature, cochlear and pupillary reflexes, galvanic skin responses, salivation, and GI activity. According to imagery advocates, people with strong imaginations, including those who can literally worry themselves sick, are excellent candidates for using imagery.

Meditation

Meditation reduces stress, which, in turn, results in decreased oxygen consumption, heart rate, and respiratory rate, and also leads to improved mood and a feeling of calmness. The most common form of meditation, called *concentrative meditation*, involves focusing on an object to eliminate distractions in the mind. The focus in a meditative exercise may be a repetitive sound (such as a word, phrase, or simple musical tune), a peaceful imaginary scenario, or the body itself, as in concentrated deep rhythmic

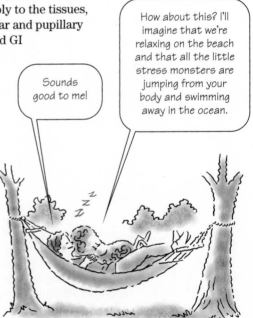

Sounds good to me!

How about this? I'll imagine that we're relaxing on the beach and that all the little stress monsters are jumping from your body and swimming away in the ocean.

Advice from the experts

Relaxation breathing

Relaxation breathing can increase lung capacity from the usual 15% to about 80% during the exercise. With daily practice, relaxation breathing and the resulting improvement in lung capacity can become automatic.

In with the good

To practice relaxation breathing, inhale through your nose but don't expand your chest. If your chest is expanding, you're breathing shallowly and actually constricting your lungs. When inhaling, your chest should remain unchanged but you should expand your belly. Imagine there's a balloon in your stomach and your job is to blow as much air into it as possible.

Inhalation should take about 6 seconds. For comparison, people typically inhale for only about 2 seconds. Inhaling more slowly brings more oxygen into the lungs.

Intermission

After inhaling, pause and hold your breath for a few seconds. Pausing exercises your diaphragm and internal muscles. When you first start doing relaxation breathing, you may feel a little out of breath from the pausing. If you feel uncomfortable, you can skip the pauses for now and insert them when you've become more comfortable with the basic pattern of inhaling and exhaling.

Out with the bad

Next, exhale slowly and evenly for 6 seconds by relaxing the abdomen and allowing the lungs to expel the air. The chest may expand slightly at this point.

Be aware that when you're practicing relaxation breathing as a conscious exercise, you should breathe through your mouth gently, not forcefully. When breathing this way during normal activity, exhale through your nose.

Putting it all together

Using this breathing technique, take 10 full, deep breaths. Inhale for 6 seconds, and then exhale for 6 seconds in a steady rhythm. After you learn the technique, there shouldn't be any pauses between inhalation and exhalation. If you have trouble with a 6-second cycle, find a cycle that's comfortable for you, such as a 3-second cycle, and gradually work your way up to 6 seconds.

Set aside 5 minutes three times each day to practice. If possible, practice your breathing while sitting comfortably in a chair with your feet flat on the floor and your arms resting loosely in your lap.

breathing. (See *Relaxation breathing.*) The focus may also be a *mantra,* a word or phrase repeated over and over in a melodic rhythm.

Focusing on an object or thought of some kind prevents the undisciplined mind from flitting from subject to subject. As you grow in experience with meditation, you'll find it easier to prolong and sustain concentration.

Let it go — the stress, that is

Another form of meditation involves "letting go" or "going with the flow" to become more sensitive to your environment. To do this, you need to be in a quiet, serene place, such as the shore, the woods, or a quiet place at home. Assume a comfortable position, such as the famous Lotus position or a similar meditative pose.

Exercise your mind

Visualization

Visualization is similar to meditation except that in visualization you're guiding your thoughts toward a set of specific images. Visualization can take many forms, but a common one involves focusing on being in a quiet, safe place.

Setting

To perform visualization, go to a quiet area with as few distractions as possible. Sit comfortably in a chair, and take at least 10 natural breaths. Close your eyes gently, and imagine the inside of your eyelids as a movie screen. Picture a physical setting that makes you feel calm and relaxed, such as a sunny clearing in the woods, a canoe ride on a still lake at sunrise, or a book-lined study with classical music playing in the background.

Colors and smells

Now sharpen your image of this place by using all of your senses to provide reality. See the flowers along the edge of the clearing. Feel the moisture in the morning mist. Listen to each note as the bassoons play off the sounds of the violins.

Sharpen the images with even more specific detail. What kind of trees are surrounding you? Are they old-growth or young trees? Is the clearing near a lake or stream? Can you hear the rushing water? Put as much detail as possible into your image.

Focus

As you work on the clarity of the vision, pay attention to your feelings. Focus on your sense of calm and restfulness. Let all the elements of the scene wash over your emotions. Remember your "place" when you finish your visualization session. When you visualize next, return to your place and add detail. Change its characteristics, if you like. Practice going to your quiet place on demand.

Take some deep breaths, relaxing your body a little more each time you exhale.

Allow your thoughts to flow from one to the other without attempting to manipulate them. (See *Visualization.*) Allow your distractions to be played out in your mind until you can gently bring your attention back to a calm, peaceful state. The aim of this sort of meditation is to lose self-consciousness and not to think in the perspective of "I."

Caring for your mind

Nearly every cultural tradition has techniques for promoting relaxation and reducing stress. You can turn your mind toward relaxation rather than stress and anxiety by controlling negative thoughts and building social supports.

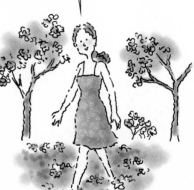

This looks like the perfect place for meditation.

Controlling negative thoughts

Some stress can be accentuated by imagining the worst possible scenario. The imagination can be highly creative. It can veer off in frightening directions if allowed to do so, creating images and events that increase anxiety.

You've got to accentuate the positive...

Positive, creative imagery can have a suggestive effect that starts the mind moving toward a goal and weakens or overcomes negative images. By imagining what goals you want to reach and visualizing how you'll achieve each goal, you can replace negative thoughts with positive ones. (See *The power of positive thinking*.) If you imagine failure, you're more likely to fail; if you imagine success, you're more likely to succeed.

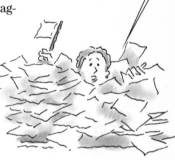

I'm accentuating the positive. I'm positively swamped!

...and eliminate the negative

To rid yourself of negative thoughts, find a quiet place, sit or lie down, close your eyes, and imagine your body as being two-dimensional with the interior completely dark. Slowly begin to inhale and exhale. Think of each exhalation as forcing some of the interior darkness from your body. Inhale and exhale the darkness until you feel that the interior of your body is no longer dark. You'll soon begin to feel the stress disappearing with each exhalation.

Another technique involves stopping yourself each time your inner voice says something negative. Replace these thoughts with positive thoughts or a mantra. You may have to repeat these

Exercise your mind

The power of positive thinking

If you plan to succeed and you visualize yourself succeeding, then you're more likely to ultimately succeed. Nurture your power of positive thinking by using these techniques:
• Psych yourself up for important events. Think about the upcoming situation, and visualize it as being a successful experience.
• Talk to yourself in a positive manner. Think of yourself as "The little engine that could." Repeat over and over, "I know I can. I know I can."

• Prepare properly. Develop a plan of action as well as contingency or alternative plans in case circumstances change.
• Label an upcoming event that could cause undue tension as a positive learning experience.
• Look at examinations and other potentially stressful events as opportunities to prove yourself by showing others what you know or what you can do. Avoid looking at these events as tests of what you don't know or can't do. Viewing them as positive opportunities can give you a feeling of power and accomplishment.

thoughts several times until you conquer your anxiety, but gradually it may help you to eliminate angry or frightening thoughts.

Building social supports

A strong social network can help control and improve a person's ability to respond effectively to stress. Social networks can take many forms, including:

- family
- friends
- peers at work
- fellow students
- religious groups
- people with shared interests, such as sports, hobbies, or social causes.

These social supports give you an outlet for discussing problems with people who care for you and want to help you. Discussing stress-producing problems can also give you new perspectives on chronic problems. Some people find that prayer can provide quiet time and help focus priorities so they can better deal with stress-provoking situations.

Asking for help

Stress is a normal part of daily life. Most of the time, the stressful situation passes or we're able to deal with it in a way that makes it manageable. At some point in our lives, however, most of us experience stress that's overwhelming. When stress interferes with your ability to do what you need — or want — to do, it's easy to feel helpless or even hopeless.

Reach out

When stress gets to that point and you can't manage it effectively, it may be time to ask for help. Help comes in many forms — from family and friends, or from professionals, such as counselors, social workers, clergy, or community-based support groups. Remember that asking for help isn't a sign of weakness; it's a sign of strength and wisdom.

If asking for help is a sign of strength, then I must be the strongest woman in the world! HELP!!!

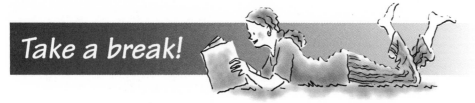

Take a break!

Destress zone

Find your way out of this stress maze and into a warm, soothing bubble bath! Watch out for roadblocks along the way that can slow you down! Check out the next page for the correct trail!

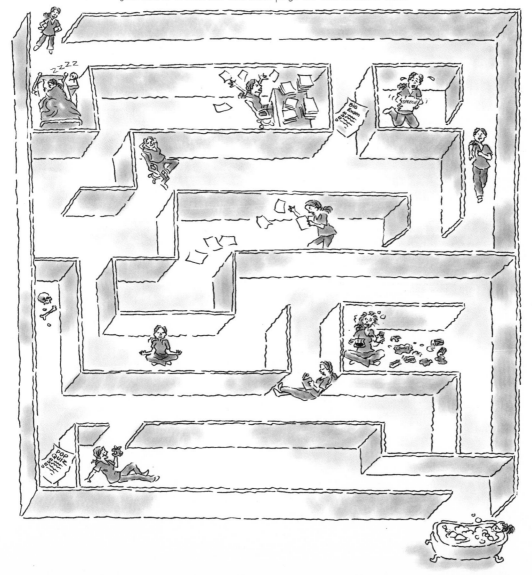

Answer key

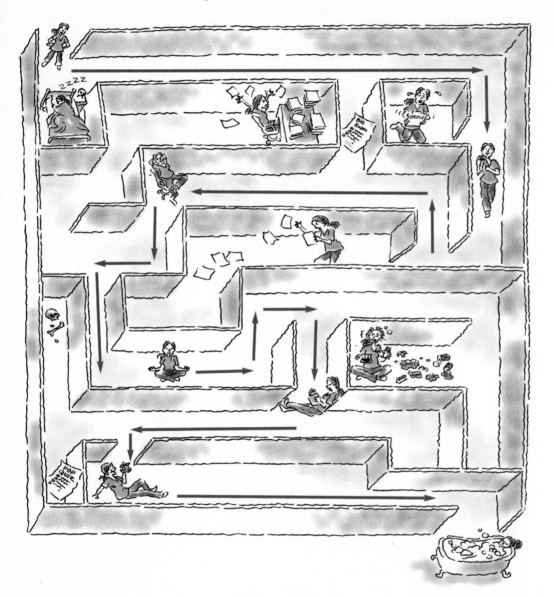

Part III Are you ready for patient care?

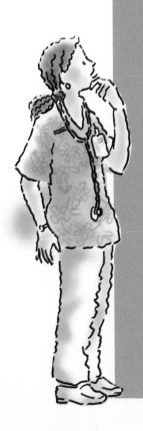

Prepping for clinical

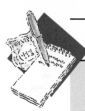

Just the facts

In this chapter, you'll learn:

♦ how to prepare for your clinical experience

♦ ways to improve your clinical skills

♦ how to meet your clinical instructor's expectations

♦ basic safety procedures to protect you and your patients

♦ about clinical evaluations and student externships.

Putting your best foot forward

> As your skills grow, you'll start seeing patients with more serious circumstances.

The experience you get during your clinical rotation at the facility helps you learn the skills you'll need to become a registered nurse. At first, you'll be assigned to meet the basic needs of patients with uncomplicated problems. Then, as your skills and confidence grow, you'll care for patients with more complex needs.

Entering the facility for a clinical rotation and caring for patients for the first time is one of the most difficult obstacles a student nurse must overcome. New situations that require you to put your skills into practice can be intimidating. It helps to remember that your clinical instructor will be there at all times to help and guide you through this experience. This chapter will also help; it provides important information to help you prepare for clinical, and grow from this experience.

Mental preparation

Clinical day is finally here. You've been learning new procedures in the skills laboratory. You've practiced these skills on mannequins, fellow nursing students, and even family, and you've been tested on them in the laboratory. Now you're ready to perform them on a patient for the first time.

It's normal to feel nervous and anxious. You're taking a big step in your nursing career. Remember that you aren't alone! Your clinical instructor is there to help you through this experience, and you can take steps to be prepared.

Applying what you've learned to a real patient is a big step! It's normal to be a bit nervous — and excited!

Dealing with anxiety

Most students feel anxious the first time they talk with a patient or perform skills, such as giving a bath, making a bed, or administering an injection. It's normal to feel this way. Sharing your concerns and fears with a few trusted classmates may help relieve some of your initial anxieties; you'll probably find out that they feel the same way too!

A little anxiety probably won't affect your clinical performance or be noticed by the patient, but high levels of anxiety interfere with your ability to learn. To help relieve anxiety, try some of the strategies presented in chapter 6 to help you relax. You can also make an appointment to see your clinical instructor or advisor. She can reassure you that what you're feeling is normal, and can help you identify your anxieties and develop a plan to reduce them. For instance, if the thought of interviewing a patient is making you anxious, review this skill in your nursing textbook. Then practice on as many people as you can until you feel comfortable. Many colleges also have counseling services that can help you cope with the stress of school and life.

Planning your time

Being a student nurse is demanding and places severe restraints on your time and energy, especially after you start your clinical rotations. There are, however, things you can do to ease some of the burden.

A little help from your friends

Most students enlist their family and friends to help get them through nursing school. Speak candidly with your family and friends about the severe limitations on your time. Tell them that, while you're in school, you won't be able to spend as much time with them as usual; this will help prevent misunderstandings. Make sure friends know that their friendship is still important, but that when school is in session you'll have less time for social activities.

Share your dirty laundry

Try to plan ahead. For instance, if you have children, you'll need to find child care that starts earlier on clinical days. Accept offers from family and friends to prepare meals, help children with homework, or do your laundry.

> Accept all offers to have others cook for you. It gives you time to study... and it tastes pretty good, too!

Learning new skills

New skills that you'll need to perform on patients in clinical are first taught in the skills laboratory at school. Skills may be learned by watching the laboratory instructor demonstrate or watching a videotape or computer simulation. To get the most out of these skills sessions, first read the procedure in your skills textbook.

A leap of faith — and practice!

The best way to learn a new skill is to leap in and practice it. You may feel awkward at first but you'll soon find that, with repetition, new skills become easier to perform. Your skills laboratory will have all the equipment you need to practice these new skills.

The search for willing victims

You may practice skills on a life-size manikin or on other nursing students. By the end of nursing school, you and your classmates will know each other very well! Skills, such as physical assessment, can be practiced on willing roommates, spouses, children, and friends. Skills involving needles and syringes will need to be practiced in the supervised skills laboratory.

> Need to practice the skills you've learned? Classmates, friends, and family members are usually more than willing to help. You never know until you ask!

Some schools require students to buy a skills kit that contains some of the common supplies that you'll need for the skills laboratory. The contents of the kit vary depending on the skills required for the particular course.

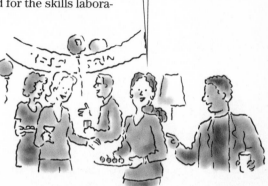

Many nursing programs require you to demonstrate a skill in the skills laboratory before you can perform it in the clinical setting. You may have a skills card that must be "signed off" by the laboratory instructor before your clinical instructor will allow you to perform the skill in the clinical setting.

If your instructor posts the patient assignment the day before clinical, check the patient's chart to see what skills you may need to perform. Then, go to the skills laboratory to practice these skills or read up on the skills in your skills textbook.

Practice makes perfect...eventually

Most schools have times when the skills laboratory is open to practice, with a laboratory instructor or student mentor available to help you if you have questions. If you have difficulty with a particular skill in clinical, your instructor may suggest or require that you go to the skills laboratory to practice some more.

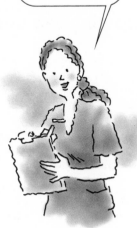

When in doubt about your appearance for your clinical rotation, always err on the side of a professional look.

Personal appearance

When you put on your nurse's uniform and student nurse badge, you'll be treated and expected to behave in a professional manner.

Uniforms

An appropriate uniform is a must for every nurse. Before you purchase a uniform, check your student handbook for specific guidelines on what vendor to use and what to buy. Usually, the vendor will come to the school at the beginning of the semester with samples of approved uniforms in different sizes to try on and order.

Dressed for success

Following a few simple guidelines will help ensure that you present yourself (and are treated) in a professional manner:
• Be clean and free from offensive odors; practice good personal hygiene and avoid wearing perfumes and scented products that might irritate or annoy patients or coworkers.
• Arrange your hair so it isn't hanging loose, and neatly trim any facial hair (mustaches and beards).
• Keep fingernails clean and trimmed, and make sure nail polish is a pale color and in good repair (without chipping). Check the policy of your clinical facility to determine whether acrylic nails and tips are permitted.
• Wear your student name tag in a prominent place at all times.
• Avoid chewing gum.
• Keep your uniform washed and pressed.
• Choose durable, comfortable, and supportive white shoes. Check with your school and facility to see if clogs or white sneakers are allowed.
• Wear makeup in moderation.
• Limit jewelry to a simple ring or wedding band, and a necklace worn inside the uniform. Limit earrings to small studs, and check your school and facility policy on the number of earrings that may be worn in each ear (typically, there's a one or two stud per ear limit). Remove any body jewelry and cover any tattoos.

When in Rome...

If the clinical facility has a more stringent dress code than your school, you must adhere to those stricter guidelines during your clinical rotation. Additional dress restrictions may be required to maintain infection control in specific areas of the facility, such as the neonatal nursery or operating room. Your clinical instructor will tell you about facility or unit dress codes during your clinical orientation.

Make sure that you wear your student nurse badge at all times, clearly identifying yourself as a student nurse and the school you're from. Your school may also require that you sew a school patch on your uniform.

You may be allowed to wear a laboratory coat over your street clothes when you're in the facility for activities that don't require direct patient contact, such as getting your clinical assignment and reviewing your patient's chart. Make sure you're dressed appropriately in professional attire—not casual clothes, such as shorts, jeans, sandals, and halter tops.

Remember, your clinical instructor has the last word on your appearance. If you aren't dressed or groomed appropriately, you may be asked to leave the clinical area.

Equipment

Your school will provide you with a list of equipment you'll need for your clinical rotation. This list may include:
• a watch with a second hand for counting your patient's heart rate and respiratory rate
• black pens for writing in the patient's chart
• a penlight for assessing pupils
• stainless steel bandage scissors for cutting tape and bandages
• a good stethoscope with a bell and diaphragm to listen to heart, lung, and bowel sounds. (Although other pieces of equipment can be obtained cheaply, the stethoscope isn't the place to skimp; spend your money on a high-quality stethoscope.)

The simple life

Some programs require students to purchase a Personal Data Assistant (PDA). Software for the PDA can take the place of a drug book, medical-surgical textbook, and other references, and the PDA is more compact and lighter weight, making it easier than books to carry to clinical. PDAs also have functions that can simplify your life, such as a calculator, date book, address book, to-do list, and memo pad.

Getting to know your instructor

Believe it or not, your clinical instructors are people too! Each instructor has her own personality. Try not to listen to stories about the instructor from other students. Keep an open mind and form your own opinions.

What's in a name?

Your instructor will let you know how she prefers to be addressed. Some prefer to be addressed by title, such as Mr., Mrs., or Dr.; others are comfortable with using first names. Whichever name your instructor prefers, it's up to you to show respect. Treat your instructor with respect, and she'll treat you with respect.

Getting to know all about you

Try to get to know your clinical instructor. For example, ask your instructor how she got into nursing, where she went to school, and positions she has held. Your instructor has a wealth of knowledge to share if you take the initiative.

Any clinical instructor will be pleased to have a student who has reviewed procedures in advance and is eager to learn. Ask questions when you're unsure. Come to clinical with the proper equipment and reference books, such as nursing care plan and drug books. It's up to you to make the most of the clinical experience. Your job is to learn all you can from it.

Nip it in the bud!

If you feel things aren't going well in your relationship with your clinical instructor, make an appointment to discuss your concerns. If the two of you can't resolve the issue by discussing it, follow the procedures outlined in your student handbook to resolve grievances.

Learning the ropes

Learning the ropes of nursing involves more than patient care. Get ready to round up some knowledge about policies and procedures, patient rights, and safety.

Your knowledge about caring for patients sets the foundation for a successful nursing career. However, being skilled in patient care is only part — albeit an essential one — of what will make you an effective nurse. Whether you'll be working in a hospital or another type of facility, each facility has its own way of doing things. The best — and most efficient — nurses learn as much as they can about how their particular facility operates. Doing so will help you provide the best possible care to your patients and you will be viewed by your colleagues as a respected professional.

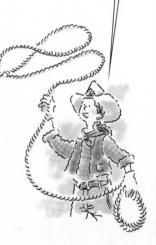

Clinical orientation

Clinical orientation typically takes place at the facility where you'll be doing your clinical rotation. It typically includes a welcome from a representative of the facility, followed by information, such as the mission statement, fire and safety policies, other emergency procedures, standard precautions, and confidentiality rules. If you need computer access, orientation also may include computer classes and assignments of passwords.

Your instructor will explain her expectations for the clinical rotation. She'll give you a schedule with the dates of the clinical experiences and times, and she'll explain written assignments and due dates. Clinical objectives and evaluation procedures will also be reviewed. Be sure to ask questions if you don't fully understand what's being explained.

Details, details

Be sure to ask where students may park. The last thing you want at the end of your clinical day is to find a parking ticket on your car or, even worse, no car at all (because it has been towed)!

Clarify whom to call if you'll be absent and by what time the call should be made. Some instructors will have you call them, whereas others may have you call the clinical unit. Missing clinical is highly discouraged and you'll likely be required to make up the missed days.

Sometimes a clinical instructor will give you a list of commonly used supplies. Treat this like a scavenger hunt and don't give up until you find everything. If you don't find what you need, ask your instructor and staff members to help you.

Patient assignment

Patients may be assigned the day before or the day of clinical. If you receive your patient assignment the day before clinical, the instructor will expect you to review the patient's chart and look up the medical diagnosis and medications. Use your nursing skills book to review the treatments you must give, and practice skills that you're unsure of in the skills laboratory. Your instructor may also require that you complete a written nursing care plan before providing nursing care.

Precare briefing

Whether you receive your assignment the day before or the day of clinical, the day commonly starts with a *preconference*. If you haven't received your patient assignment, your instructor will give it to you during this time. If you received your assignment the previous day, your instructor will expect you to briefly discuss your care plan for your patient and your priorities for patient care. This is also a time to ask questions about your assignment.

Your clinical instructor will select patients to help you meet your clinical objectives. In your first clinical assignments, your instructor will choose patients who aren't too sick for you to meet their needs. As you progress, your clinical instructor will seek patients that will challenge you.

Postscript

At the end of the clinical day, students meet with the instructor for a *postconference*. This meeting is a time to discuss patient problems and student concerns and apply classroom content to actual patient care or case studies provided by your instructor.

Policies and procedures

Every health care facility has *policies* — a set of general principles that guide care. From these policies flow the *procedures*, which describe the specific way a task should be accomplished. Policies and procedures set the standards for the performance of nursing care.

Each facility's unit has policy and procedure manuals. Know where these manuals are located and refer to them often. Even though you may have learned a certain way of performing a skill, the procedure at your clinical facility may be different. When you're practicing at a facility, you must adhere to its policies, procedures, and protocols, which may also be found on the facility's computer system.

HIPAA

The *Health Insurance Portability and Accountability Act (HIPAA)* protects the privacy, confidentiality, and security of all medical information. Only those who have a need to know patient information in order to provide care for the patient and those authorized by the patient to have access to information can lawfully receive oral, written, or electronic information. During your clinical orientation, you'll receive information about maintaining patient rights under HIPAA that's specifically tailored to the health care facility. Failure to comply with HIPAA, intentionally or unintentionally, could result in criminal or civil penalties. (See *Patient rights under HIPAA*.)

Some safeguards you must practice during patient care to maintain privacy include:
• protecting your computer password and logging off the computer when you're finished
• keeping patients' charts closed when not in use

Patient rights under HIPAA

The goal of the Health Insurance Portability and Accountability Act (HIPAA) is to provide safeguards against the inappropriate use and release of personal medical information, including all medical records and identifiable health information in any form (electronic, paper, and verbal). Patients are the beneficiaries of this privacy rule, which includes these six rights:

right to give consent before information is released for treatment, payment, or health care operations

right to be educated about the provider's policy on privacy protection

right to access their medical records

right to request that their medical records be amended for accuracy

right to access the history of nonroutine disclosures (disclosures that didn't occur in the course of treatment, payment, or health care operations or those not specifically authorized by the patient)

right to request that the provider restrict the use and routine disclosure of information he has. (Providers aren't required to grant this request, especially if they think the information is important to the quality of patient care such as disclosing human immunodeficiency virus status to another medical provider who's providing treatment.)

• not leaving faxes and computer printouts unattended
• disposing of unneeded patient information (such as your report sheets) in special receptacles before you leave the facility
• not discussing patient information for purposes other than learning (this includes not discussing such information with your family and friends)
• avoiding discussing patient information with visitors unless they're cleared by the patient
• not posting your patient's name near his door
• keeping your voice down when talking about the patient with other health care workers — on the telephone or in person
• removing identifying information before handing in written class work, such as a nursing care plan.

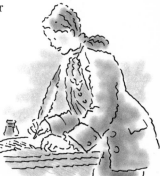

Patients are more involved in their health care than ever before. Patients' rights bills have helped reinforce their expectation of quality care.

Patient's Bill of Rights

In 1977, the National League for Nursing (NLN) published a patient's bill of rights. It states that the NLN believes nurses are responsible for upholding these rights of patients:

• People have the right to health care that's accessible and that meets professional standards, regardless of the setting.

• Patients have the right to courteous and individualized health care that is equitable, humane, and given without discrimination as to race, color, creed, sex, national origin, source of payment, or ethical or political beliefs.

• Patients have the right to information about their diagnosis, prognosis, and treatment—including alternatives to care and risks involved—in terms they and their families can readily understand, so that they can give their informed consent.

• Patients have the legal right to informed participation in all decisions concerning their health care.

• Patients have the right to information about the qualifications, names, and titles of personnel responsible for providing their health care.

• Patients have the right to refuse observation by those not directly involved in their care.

• Patients have the right to privacy during interview, examination, and treatment.

• Patients have the right to privacy in communicating and visiting with persons of their choice.

• Patients have the right to refuse treatments, medications, or participation in research and experimentation, without punitive action being taken against them.

• Patients have the right to coordination and continuity of health care.

• Patients have the right to appropriate instruction or education from health care personnel so that they can achieve an optimal level of wellness and an understanding of their basic health needs.

• Patients have the right to confidentiality of all records (except as otherwise provided for by law or third-party payer contracts) and all communications, written or oral, between patients and health care providers.

• Patients have the right of access to all health records pertaining to them, the right to challenge and to have their records corrected for accuracy, and the right to transfer of all such records in the case of continuing care.

• Patients have the right to information on the charges for services, including the right to challenge these.

• Above all, patients have the right to be fully informed as to all their rights in all health care settings.

Reprinted from a 1977 publication with permission from the National League for Nursing.

Patient rights

Patients are more knowledgeable, assertive, and involved in their health care than ever before. They question their diagnoses, seek assurances that their treatment is appropriate, and take action when care doesn't meet their expectations. They demand more education about wellness-related issues, risks, alternatives, and benefits before consenting to treatment. In addition, patients expect confidentiality to be maintained. Bills of rights for patients have helped to reinforce the public's expectation of quality care. (See *Patient's Bill of Rights*.)

As a student nurse, you need to uphold these patient rights as you plan and provide care. Become familiar with the facility's policy on patient rights. View your patient as a partner in the health care process. In planning your patient's care, recognize his right to participate in decisions. Help your patient set realistic goals for his health care and teach him the various approaches he can use to achieve them.

Safety

One of the most important concerns of your clinical instructor is maintaining a safe environment—for your patient and you.

Patient safety

Patient safety is the responsibility of all members of the health care team—including you. Be sure to familiarize yourself with the facility's policies and procedures concerning safety. If you're unsure, then ask; always err on the side of caution.

Safety concerns will vary according to facility type and your patient's capabilities and needs. You can, however, take basic steps to reduce your patient's risk.

Patient falls

Because almost anything can cause a fall—improper transfer, medication, inappropriate use of bed rails, debris on the floor, or out-of-place equipment—be vigilant and protective of your patients. (See *Preventing falls*.)

Restraints

A *restraint* is used to physically restrict a patient's freedom of movement and normal access to his body. Use restraints only if your patient is at risk for harming himself or others and when other less restrictive measures haven't worked. Restraints are considered a last resort because they can cause many problems, including limited mobility, skin breakdown, impaired circulation, loss of bowel and bladder control, psychological distress, and strangulation. (See *Alternatives to restraints*, page 144.)

Equipment safety

You're responsible for making sure the equipment you use for patient care is free from defects. You're also responsible for using all equipment properly, according to the instructions and the procedure manual. If you have questions about equipment use, ask your instructor.

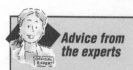
Advice from the experts

Preventing falls

Almost anything can cause a patient to fall, particularly if he's elderly or receiving medication. Here are some ways to prevent falls:
• Make sure his bed's side rails are kept up, when indicated.
• Orient him to his surroundings and to the time, and reorient him as necessary.
• Provide adequate lighting and a clean, clutter-free area.
• Review the medications that may increase his risk of falling.
• Monitor regularly.
• Offer a bedpan or commode regularly.
• Make sure that adequate staff is available to perform safe patient transfers to or from the bed, and to assist the patient as needed.
• Make sure that the patient wears proper shoes for walking.
• See that the call light is within easy reach and is in working condition.
• Supervise the patient when he's in a chair.

Alternatives to restraints

Restraints must be used only as a last resort after all other measures have failed to keep a patient from harming himself or others. They should be applied in the least restrictive manner and for as short a time as possible.

Risk reduction

To reduce the need for restraints, take an individualized approach that seeks to prevent behavior problems. Look for an underlying problem that may be causing your patient's behavior—such as adverse drug effects, infection, electrolyte imbalance, or hypoxia—and take measures to correct the problem.

Look for *"agenda behaviors"* in which the patient's behavior may be an attempt to correct a problem, such as pain, hunger, fatigue, heat, cold, or the need for toileting.

Create an environment that's free from restraints and encourages patient mobility. Creating such an environment requires unit and facility commitment because policy changes and even structural changes may be required.

Options available

If the problem behavior continues after you've identified and corrected conditions that may be the cause, consider alternatives to restraints, such as:
• reorienting the patient as needed
• providing explanations for procedures
• keeping the patient warm, dry, and comfortable
• establishing eye contact and talking to the patient
• listening to and validating the patient's concerns
• determining the patient's routines and habits and trying to accommodate them
• wrapping elastic compression bandages around I.V. sites, other tubing, or dressings
• switching to a capped I.V. line, if possible
• determining whether equipment or treatment is really necessary
• moving tubing or equipment out of the patient's sight
• using an abdominal binder to cover abdominal drains, tubes, dressings, and urinary catheters.

Disease transmission

To reduce the risk of transmitting a disease to your patients, wash your hands! Proper hand washing (with soap and water or waterless soap) is the single most effective thing you can do to prevent the spread of infection. (See *Proper hand-washing technique.*)

Personal safety

While providing safe care to your patients, you also must protect yourself. As in patient safety, prevention is key when protecting yourself on the clinical unit.

Infection

To protect yourself from infection, all blood and other body fluids, tissues, and contact with mucous membranes and broken skin

Proper hand-washing technique

To minimize the spread of infection, follow these basic hand-washing instructions.

With your hands angled downward under the faucet, adjust the water temperature until it's comfortably warm.

Work up a generous lather by scrubbing vigorously for 10 seconds. Be sure to clean beneath your fingernails, around your knuckles, and along the sides of your fingers and hands. Rinse your hands completely to wash away suds and microorganisms. Pat your hands dry with a paper towel.

To prevent recontamination on your hands, cover each faucet handle with a paper towel before turning off the water.

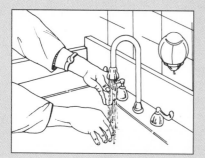
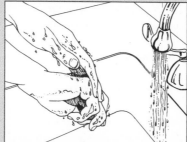
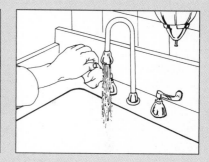

should be handled as if they contain infectious organisms, regardless of your patient's diagnosis or appearance. Follow standard precautions at all times. This includes wearing gloves if you may be in contact with blood or other body fluids, tissue, mucous membranes, and nonintact skin. (See *Standard precautions*, page 146.)

A safety fashion statement

If a procedure may result in splashing or splattering of blood or other body fluids on the face, wear a mask and goggles or face shield. If the procedure may result in splashing or splattering of blood on the body, wear a fluid-resistant gown or apron.

Handle needles and sharp equipment carefully, and immediately place them in special *sharps containers* after use. (Your instructor will point out these containers during orientation to the unit.) Most facilities use syringes and I.V. equipment with safety features that reduce the risk of getting stuck. Practice handling this equipment before using it on a patient.

Advice from the experts

Standard precautions

These guidelines were developed by the Centers for Disease Control and Prevention (CDC) to provide the widest possible protection against the transmission of infection. CDC officials recommend that health care workers handle all blood and other body fluids, tissues, and contact with mucous membranes and broken skin as if they contained infectious agents, regardless of the patient's diagnosis, and take these precautions:

• Wash your hands before and after patient care, after removing gloves, or immediately after contamination with blood, body fluid, excretions, secretions, or drainage.

• Wear gloves if you will or could come in contact with blood or other body fluids, specimens, tissue, secretions, excretions, mucous membranes, broken skin, or contaminated objects or surfaces.

• Change gloves and wash your hands between patients; when caring for the same patient, change gloves and wash your hands if you touch anything with a high concentration of microorganisms.

• Wear a fluid-resistant gown, eye protection, and a mask during procedures that are likely to generate droplets of blood or body fluids.

• Carefully handle used patient care equipment that's soiled with blood or body fluids; follow facility guidelines for cleaning and disinfecting equipment and environmental surfaces.

• Keep contaminated linens away from your body and place in properly labeled containers.

• Handle needles and sharps carefully and immediately discard in an impervious disposal box after use; use sharps with safety features whenever possible.

• Immediately notify your supervisor of a needle-stick or sharp-instrument injury, mucosal splash, or contamination of nonintact skin with blood or other body fluids to initiate appropriate investigation of the incident and care.

• Use mouthpieces, resuscitation bags, or ventilation devices in place of mouth-to-mouth resuscitation.

• Place a patient in a private room if he can't maintain hygiene measures or may contaminate the environment.

• If occupational exposure to blood is likely, get the hepatitis B vaccine series.

• Become familiar with your facility's infection control policies and procedures.

Accidents happen!

Immediately notify your clinical instructor if you receive a needle-stick or sharp instrument injury, splashing on any of your mucous membranes, or contamination of broken skin with blood or other body fluids. Your instructor will assist you in immediate first aid, fill out an incident report, and guide you to receive the proper follow-up care. Because of the risk of occupational exposure to hepatitis B, many schools require you to get the hepatitis B vaccine series.

> Protective gear may not be glamorous, but neither is contracting an infectious disease from a patient.

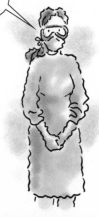

Back injuries

Back injuries are the most common physical reason nurses lose time from work. Many patient care activities require you to push, pull, lift, and carry. By using proper body mechanics, you can avoid back injuries and reduce the risk of injuring the patient as well. Correct body mechanics can be summed up as three principles:

Keep a low center of gravity by flexing your hips and knees instead of bending at the waist. This position distributes weight evenly between your upper and lower body and helps maintain balance.

Create a wide base of support by spreading your feet apart. This tactic provides lateral stability and lowers your body's center of gravity.

Maintain proper body alignment and keep your body's center of gravity directly over the base of support by moving your feet rather than twisting and bending at the waist.

Chemical injuries

Many potentially hazardous chemicals are routinely used in health care facilities. Chemotherapy drugs, radiation, and powerful cleaning solutions and disinfectants are common hazards. A *Material Safety Data Sheet (MSDS)* provides you with information about the physical and chemical hazards that can occur from these substances. Each MSDS provides information about the chemicals found in a substance and how to treat exposure to that substance. Each unit will have an MSDS manual. Make sure you know its location on your clinical unit.

Getting to know the staff

During clinical orientation, your instructor will take you on a tour of the nursing unit and introduce you to the various staff members, including the clinical nurse-manager, nurses, unit secretary, cleaning staff, nursing assistant, physical therapist, respiratory therapist, dietitian, pharmacist, and volunteers.

Part of your clinical experience will be learning the various roles of the members of the health care team as well as learning to work with many different personalities. You'll learn that each person has her own unique talents and skills. Work to develop and maintain a positive, upbeat attitude and realize that you have much to learn from every member of the staff. Show respect for each member of the team and for the job they do. Showing respect is the best way to ensure that you'll be treated with respect in return.

Accountability

As a student nurse, you're accountable for your actions. This means you're responsible for your behaviors and decisions in providing care to your patients. While you're providing nursing care, you're held to the same standard of care as a registered nurse.

When in doubt, ask!

You demonstrate accountability when you ask questions if you're unsure. Never attempt to perform a skill of which you're unsure or use a piece of equipment you haven't been taught to operate. Don't be afraid to ask for help. Your instructor is always available while you're caring for patients. The nurses and other members of the health care team will also be glad to answer your questions. Most people remember what it was like being a student and will be glad to help you!

The dog ate my homework!

Your instructor will expect you to show accountability for your learning. This includes showing up on time for clinical in a clean uniform and being prepared to care for your patient. If you're going to be absent, you demonstrate accountability by calling the designated telephone number at the appropriate time and making up the worked missed within the stated time frame. You show accountability when you communicate your concerns about assessment findings to the primary nurse and your instructor.

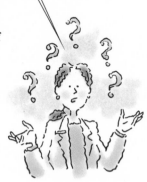

Asking questions will show your instructor that you're taking your job seriously and you want to do things right the first time around!

Knowing your patients

To truly get to know a patient, you first must establish a trusting relationship that makes the patient feel safe and respected. This kind of relationship is called a *therapeutic relationship*.

The first step in developing this relationship is to introduce yourself. Remember, the patient and his family start forming an impression about you as soon as you enter the patient's room. Begin by knocking on the patient's door before entering. This shows respect for your patient's privacy.

Hello, my name is...

Introduce yourself with confidence and a smile as you tell the patient your first and last name. Then, clearly identify yourself as a student nurse and tell your patient the name of the nursing school you're attending. Ask the patient what he would like to be called. Some patients prefer to be addressed by their first names; others are more formal and prefer that you use their title. Explain to the patient that, although you'll be providing care for the day, the registered nurse is still responsible for his overall care and will be working closely with you.

While you're providing care, talk with the patient about his perceptions of care and his fears and concerns. This discussion may provide more useful information than a formal nursing interview. Listening helps the patient feel understood, so he'll be more comfortable discussing problems.

A pleasant surprise!

You may be pleasantly surprised to learn that your patient feels fortunate to have a student nurse. Nurses are commonly busy providing care to so many patients that the one-on-one care provided by a student nurse may be extremely comforting and reassuring.

Know your patient's meds

Look up each of your patient's medications in your drug book before administering them. Make sure you know why the medication is being given, how it works, the safe dose range, adverse effects, how it's given, and any special considerations. Your instructor will be sure to ask you! (See *Medication errors*.)

When you're right, you're right!

To administer medications safely, following the *six rights of medication administration*:

Right drug — To ensure that you're giving the right medication, first check the order on the patient's medication record against the doctor's order. Then check the label on the medication *three* times before giving it.

Right patient — Confirm the patient's identity by asking his name and checking the name, room number, and medical record number on his wrist band. If the facility uses a bar code scanning system, be sure to scan your badge, the patient's wristband, and the medication's bar code.

Right time — Confirm that you're giving the medication at the right time and within the allowable time range, such as within 30 minutes before or after the scheduled time.

Right dosage — Check the dosage *three* times before giving the medication. If a dosage calculation is needed, have your instructor verify your calculations.

Right route — Check to make sure that you're giving the medication by the prescribed route.

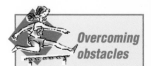

Overcoming obstacles

Medication errors

When it comes to medications, safety is priority one! If this student's question sounds familiar, see the words of wisdom for some tips.

Question

I'm nervous about making medication errors when administering medications. How can I avoid them?

Words of wisdom

• Never give a medication poured or prepared by someone else.

• Never allow the medication cart or tray out of your sight after you've prepared a dose.

• Never leave a medication at a patient's bedside — watch him swallow the medication.

• Never return unwrapped or prepared medications to the stock supply; dispose of it and notify the pharmacist.

• Keep medications locked at all times.

• Watch for similar sounding medication names, unclear orders, wrong routes of administration, and dosage miscalculations.

Right documentation — Record the time and date the medication was administered, and note adverse reactions and other pertinent information.

The homestretch

Your work will be evaluated at the end of your clinical rotation. This evaluation not only determines whether you've met the requirements of the rotation, it also helps to identify your strengths as well as areas that need improvement.

After your clinical rotation, you may choose to supplement what you've learned with a clinical externship, which provides you with additional experience, and may even help you get your "foot in the door" for your first nursing job.

Clinical evaluation

You'll need to meet specific clinical objectives by the end of the course to progress to the next level. These objectives can be found in your course syllabus. An evaluation tool is used to determine whether you've met these objectives. Although these objectives and the evaluation tool will be reviewed in the course orientation, you should review the objectives and evaluate your performance each week to make sure you're on the right track. (See *Areas of clinical evaluation.*)

Two types of evaluations may be used. A *formative evaluation* gives you weekly or mid-semester feedback. It helps you identify your strengths and weaknesses so you can make adjustments to be successful in the course. A *summative evaluation* is performed at the end of the clinical experience to determine whether you've met the course objectives (in other words, whether you've passed the course!).

You and your instructor will fill out evaluation forms and meet to discuss your progress, strengths, and weaknesses. If you're having difficulty with your clinical performance, your instructor will work with you to develop a plan or contract for improvement. If you don't have weekly or mid-semester evaluations, you may want to schedule an appointment with your instructor to discuss your progress.

Externship

A student *externship* can provide you with work experience in a clinical setting to help you strengthen your skills and bridge the

---

Areas of clinical evaluation

An evaluation tool is used to determine whether you've met the clinical objectives for the course. Typically, you'll be evaluated in these areas:
• using the nursing process and individualizing care
• organizing and prioritizing care
• maintaining a safe environment for your patient and yourself
• demonstrating professional behaviors such as accountability
• following policies and procedures, including the Health Insurance Portability and Accountability Act
• collaborating and working with the health care team
• documenting patient care
• performing health teaching
• performing nursing skills safely
• using therapeutic communication skills.

gap between nursing school and clinical practice as an entry level nurse. As an added bonus, many facilities pay you a stipend for your participation.

To take part in an externship program, you must be enrolled as a student in an accredited nursing program. If you're in a baccalaureate program, you may enroll after you've completed your junior year. If you're in an associate degree program, you're eligible at the end of your first year of clinical experience. Some externship programs require that you maintain a certain grade point average.

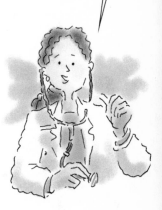

Externships give you additional clinical experience and a few bucks to boot!

How I spent my summer vacation

Some externship programs may be 8 to 12 weeks during the summer, whereas others run all year with schedules that complement your school commitment. You'll be assigned an experienced registered nurse as a preceptor on a specific clinical unit, and you'll be expected to work the preceptor's schedule. You may also rotate through other departments, such as radiology, physical therapy, and occupational therapy.

Your experience will begin with an orientation to the facility. Classroom sessions supplement the clinical experience and may include such topics as treatments, infection control, safety issues, emergency situations, documentation, communication skills, and HIPAA training. Some programs offer educational programs and skills sessions.

The right stuff

To apply for an externship, you'll need to fill out an application. You'll be asked to submit proof of cardiopulmonary resuscitation certification, immunization records, malpractice insurance, and tuberculosis screening. Many facilities ask you to include your resumé with your application. (See chapter 11 for tips on effective resumé writing.) Most facilities request two or three references, including one from your clinical instructor. Be sure to contact your references before you list them, and ask if they would be willing to provide a reference for you. Never list someone as a reference without first asking their permission.

During your externship program, your skills, enthusiasm, and ability to work as a member of a team will be observed. If your performance has been favorable, the nurse-manager may offer you a job after graduation. You benefit by gaining new skills and confidence, and the facility benefits by being able to recruit staff and reduce the amount of orientation required for a new graduate nurse.

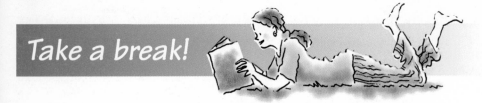

Take a break!

Prepping for patients

Get ready! Your clinical experience involves a series of steps that prepare you for your first patient assignment as a new nurse. It doesn't happen magically on the day you arrive at the facility.

To help you prepare, place these steps that relate to preparing for your clinical experience in proper sequence by numbering them from 1 to 10. Reviewing these steps before clinical will help you prepare for patient care before you even step into the patient's room. Answers below.

_____ 1. Eat a good breakfast on the morning of clinical.

_____ 2. Reevaluate the priorities of care for your patient based on additional information that you've received about the patient.

_____ 3. Perform the practice skills in the skills laboratory. Perform interviews and assessments on classmates, friends, or family members.

_____ 4. Take a deep breath, try to relax, and head toward your patient's room.

_____ 5. The night before, put out your uniform, watch, socks, shoes, bandage scissors, penlight, stethoscope, books, notebook, black pen, car keys, and your lunch money in preparation for clinical.

_____ 6. Participate in a preclinical conference; receive a nursing report from the nurse on the outgoing shift.

_____ 7. Pay close attention and take notes during the hospital orientation session.

_____ 8. Get 6 to 8 hours of sleep the night before clinical.

_____ 9. Receive your patient assignment, look up medical diagnoses and medications, and establish priorities of care.

_____ 10. Arrive at the hospital 15 to 30 minutes early.

Answer key

If your clinical instructor provides your patient assignment the morning of clinical, your answers should be in this order: 5, 9, 1, 10, 3, 8, 2, 4, 7, 6.

If your clinical instructor provides your patient assignment the day before clinical, your answers should be in this order: 6, 9, 1, 10, 4, 8, 2, 5, 3, 7.

Planning your nursing care

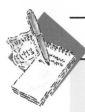

Just the facts

In this chapter, you'll learn:

♦ about common charting forms and the information they contain

♦ how to use the nursing process and nursing care plans

♦ how to apply concept mapping to your nursing care

♦ about interdisciplinary teams and how to work with them.

Making sense of the paperwork

As you prepare for your clinical day, you'll need to be familiar with the many types of paperwork found in your patient's chart.

Paper, paper everywhere!

You'll use many types of forms to gather information about your patient and to record your nursing assessments, interventions, and evaluations. (See *A close look at a medical record*, page 154.)
  Some of the more common types of paperwork you'll encounter include the:
• Kardex
• admission assessment
• medication administration record (MAR)
• flow sheets
• teaching sheets
• discharge summaries.

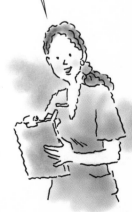

Understanding charts is a key part of your job!

Kardex

The patient care Kardex, sometimes called the *nursing Kardex*, gives you a quick overview of basic patient care information. A Kardex typically contains boxes that allow you to check off items that apply to the patient or may be a computerized printout updat-

A close look at a medical record

Although each health care facility has its own system for keeping medical records, most records contain the documents described here:

• *face sheet*—first page of the medical record; contains the patient's name, birth date, social security number, address, marital status, closest relative or guardian, food or drug allergies, admitting diagnosis, and attending doctor

• *medical history and physical examination*—completed by the doctor; contains the initial medical examination and evaluation data

• *doctor's order sheet*—a record of the doctor's medical orders

• *initial nursing assessment form*—contains nursing data, including health history and physical assessment findings

• *integrated assessment form*—used by all members of the health care team

• *problem or nursing diagnosis list*—list of the patient's problems; used with problem-oriented medical records

• *nursing care plan*—based on information gathered during the patient assessment; specifies patient's care needs, planned interventions, and the patient's progress toward meeting goals and objectives

• *graphic form*—flow sheet that tracks the patient's temperature, pulse, respiratory rate, blood pressure and, possibly, daily weight; also may record skin care, blood glucose levels, urinalysis results, neurologic assessment data, and patient intake and output; the nurse dates, initials, or checks off the appropriate column to show a task was completed

• *medication administration record*—lists medications a patient receives, including dosage, administration route, site, date, and time

• *nurses' progress notes*—details patient care information, nursing interventions, and patient responses

• *doctors' progress notes*—contains doctors' observations, notes on the patient's progress, and treatment data

• *diagnostic findings*—contains diagnostic and laboratory data

• *health care team records*—includes information from the physical therapist, respiratory therapist, social worker, and other team members

• *consultation sheets*—includes evaluations by specialists consulted for diagnostic and treatment recommendations

• *discharge plan and summary*—presents a brief account of the patient's time in the facility and plans for care after discharge.

ed by the nurse or unit clerk via the computer system. It also contains space for recording current orders for medications, patient care activities, treatments, and tests. (See *Considering the Kardex.*)

Kardex quickie

As a student, you'll find that the Kardex is a helpful overview of your patient's condition and nursing care needs. You'll want to review the Kardex before trying to wade through a lengthy chart. The Kardex tells you just about everything you'll need to know to get started with your patient care.

You'll refer to the Kardex throughout the day and during change-of-shift report. Typically, the Kardex includes:
• the patient's name, age, marital status, religion, and the admitting doctor's name
• medical diagnoses, listed by priority
• nursing diagnoses, listed by priority
• current doctors' orders for medication, treatments, diet, I.V. therapy, diagnostic tests, procedures, and other measures

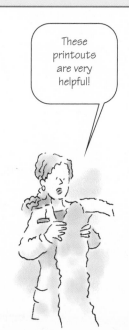

These printouts are very helpful!

Considering the Kardex

Here's an example of a patient care Kardex for a medical-surgical unit. The Kardex gives you quick access to basic patient care information. Remember that the categories, words, and phrases on a Kardex are brief and are intended to trigger images of special circumstances, procedures, activities, or patient conditions. Kardexes may be handwritten or computer generated.

Care status
Self-care ☐
Partial care with assistance ☐
Complete care ☑
Shower with assistance ☐
Tub ☐
Active exercises ☐
Passive exercises ☐

Special Care
Back care ☑
Mouth care ☑
Foot care ☐
Perineal care ☑
Catheter care ☐
Tracheostomy care ☐
Other (specify)_____ ☐

Condition
Satisfactory ☐
Fair ☐
Guarded ☑
Critical ☐
No code ☐
Advance directive?
   Yes ☑
   No ☐
Date *11/12/05*

Prosthesis
Dentures
   upper ☑
   lower ☑
Contact lenses ☐
Glasses ☑
Hearing aid ☑
Other (specify)_____ ☐

Isolation
Strict ☐
Contact ☐
Airborne ☑
Neutropenic ☐
Droplet ☐
Other (specify)_____ ☐

Diet
Type: *low-fat, no conc. sweets*
Force fluids ☐
NPO ☐
Assist with feeding ☐
Isolation tray ☑
Calorie count ☐
Supplements_____

Tube feedings ☐
Type: _____
Rate: _____
Route: _____
   NG ☐
   G tube ☐
   J tube ☐

Admission
Height: *60"*
Weight: *145 lb (61 kg)*
BP: *124/72*
TPR: *100.4 T.P.O. - 92-24*

Frequency
BP: *q 4°*
TPR: *q 4°*
Apical pulses:
Peripheral pulses: *q 4°*
Weight:
Neuro check:
Monitor:
Strips:
Turn: *q 2°*
Cough: *q 1°*
Deep breathe: *q 1°*
Central venous
   pressure:
Other (specify)_____

GI tubes
Salem sump ☐
Levin tube ☐
Feeding tube ☐
Type (specify):_____
Other (specify):_____ ☐

Activity
Bed rest ☑
Chair t.i.d. ☐
Dangle ☐
Commode ☐
Commode with assist ☐
Ambulate ☐
BRP ☐
Fall-risk category (specify): ____ ☐
Other (specify):_____ ☐

Mode of transport
Wheelchair ☐
Stretcher ☑
With oxygen ☑

I.V. devices
Saline lock ☐
Peripheral I.V. ☐
Central line ☐
Triple-lumen CVP ☑
Hickman ☐
Jugular ☐
Peripherally inserted ☐
PICC ☐
Parenteral nutrition ☐
Irrigations:_____

Dressings
Type:
Change: *CVP*
   as needed

> The check marks are intended to alert you to important patient care considerations.

(continued)

Considering the Kardex *(continued)*

Respiratory therapy
Pulse oximetry
   SvO_2 level (%)_____ ☐
Oxygen ☑
Liters/minute _10 L/min_____
Method
   Nasal cannula ☐
   Face mask ☐
   Venturi (Venti) mask ☐
   Nonrebreather mask ☐
   Trach collar ☐
Nebulizer ☐
Chest PT ☐
Incentive spirometry ☐
T-piece ☐
Ventilator ☐
   Type: _____
   Settings: _____
Other (specify)_____ ☐

Drains
Type: _____
Number: _____
Location: _____

Urine output
I&O ☑
Strain urine ☐
Indwelling catheter ☑
Date inserted _11/12/05_____
Size: ____16 Fr._____
Intermittent catheter ☐
   Frequency: _____

Side rails
Constant ☐
PRN ☐
Nights ☐

You can quickly find the information you need with this format.

Restraints
Date: _____
Type: _____

Specimens and tests
CBC daily
24-hour collection
Other (specify)_____

Stools

Special notes

Social services
consulted 11/12/05

- results of diagnostic tests and procedures
- consultations
- permitted activities, functional limitations, assistance that's needed, and safety precautions.

Admission assessment

The admission assessment — also known as the *admission database form* — is used to document your patient's initial assessment. The information on this assessment is usually broad because it's used to establish a comprehensive database.

    The style of the admission assessment may be open-ended, with preprinted headings and questions. It may also be close-ended, with preprinted headings, checklists, and questions with specific responses (you simply check off the appropriate response). Most facilities use a combination of different styles in one form.

Admission mission

A completed admission assessment can provide you with a lot of useful information about your patient, including:

- baseline data that's later used for comparison with the patient's progress
- information about the patient's current health status, and clues about actual and potential health problems (for example, prescription and over-the-counter drug use, and possible drug allergies)
- insight into your patient's ability to comply with therapy, and his expectations of treatments
- details about the patient's lifestyle, family relationships, and cultural influences. (Information about the patient's living arrangements, caregivers, resources, and support systems will be needed during discharge planning.)

Medication administration record

An MAR is used to record medication orders and document administration of those medications.

What, when, how?

The MAR tells you the medications that your patient is receiving, including the medication name and dose, the times it's being given, and the route by which it's given. The administration site is documented if the medication is given by the intradermal, subcutaneous, or I.M. route. The MAR also indicates if and why a medication wasn't given. Some facilities use a separate MAR for medications that are administered as needed.

Flow sheets

Typically, you'll find information related to physical assessment of the patient and routine aspects of patient care, such as activities of daily living (ADLs), fluid balance, nutrition, pain, and skin integrity on flow sheets. Also documented on flow sheets are specific nursing interventions, such as repositioning and turning the patient, range-of-motion (ROM) exercises, wound care, and medication administration.

Flow sheets have spaces for recording dates, times, and specific interventions. Many facilities also document I.V. therapy and patient education on flow sheets. The style and format of flow sheets may vary to fit the needs of patients on particular units. (See *Go with the flow sheets*, pages 158 and 159.)

Making your mark

The flow sheet is commonly a checklist that requires you to make a mark at a timed interval to document a pattern in a particular activity or observation. Other forms use accepted symbols or labels

(Text continues on page 160.)

Go with the flow sheets

As this example shows, a *patient care flow sheet* lets you quickly document routine interventions.

PATIENT CARE FLOW SHEET

Be sure to initial your entry.

Date: 11/22/05	2300-0700	0700-1500	1500-2300
RESPIRATORY			
Breath sounds	clear 2330 AG	Crackles LLL 0800 JM	clear 1600 HM
Treatments/Results		Nebulizer 0830 JM	
Cough/Results		Mod. amt. tenacious yellow mucus 0900 JM	
O₂ therapy	Nasal cannula @2 L/min AG	Nasal cannula @2 L/min JM	Nasal cannula @2 L/min HM
CARDIAC			
Chest pain			
Heart sounds	Normal S₁ and S₂ AG	Normal S₁ and S₂ JM	S₂ HM
Telemetry	N/A	N/A	
PAIN			
Type and location	Ⓛ flank 0400 AG	Ⓛ flank 1000 JM	Ⓛ flank 1600 HM
Intervention	meperidine 0415 AG	reposition and meperidine 1010 JM	meperidine 1615 HM
Pt response	Improved from #9 to #3 in 1/2 hour AG	Improved from #8 to #2 in 1/2 hr JM	complete relief in 1 hr HM
NUTRITION			
Type		regular JM	Regular HM
Toleration %		90% JM	80% HM
Supplement		1 can Ensure JM	
ELIMINATION			
Stool appearance			
Enema	N/A	N/A	N/A
Results			
Bowel sounds	present all quadrants 2330 AG	present all quadrants 0800 JM	hyperactive all quadrants 1600 HM
Urine appearance	clear amber 0400 AG	clear amber 1000 JM	Dark yellow 1500 HM
Indwelling urinary catheter	N/A	N/A	N/A
Catheter irrigations			

Note the exact time.

Make sure you document your patient's response to medications.

Use the flow sheet to track changes in your patient's responses.

Go with the flow sheets (continued)

PATIENT CARE FLOW SHEET

Date 11/22/05	2300-0700	0700-1500	1500-2300
TUBES			
Type	N/A	N/A	N/A
Irrigation	——	——	——
Drainage appearance	——	——	——
HYGIENE			
Self/partial/ complete	——	Partial 1000 JM	Partial 2100 HM
Oral care	——	1000 JM	2100 HM
Back care	0400 AF	1000 JM	2100 HM
Foot care	——	1000 JM	——
Remove/reapply elastic stockings	2330 AF	1000 JM	2100 HM
ACTIVITY			
Type	bed rest AF	OOB to chair x 20 min 1000 JM	OOB to chair x 20 min 1800 HM
Toleration	Turns self AF	Tol. well JM	Tol. well
Repositioned	2330 supine AF 0400 (L) side AF	(L) side 0800 JM (R) side 1200 JM	self HM
ROM	——	1000 (active) JM 1400 (active) JM	1800 (active) HM 2200 (active) HM
SLEEP			
Sleeps well	0400 AF 0600 AF	N/A	N/A
Awake at intervals	2300 AF 0400 AF	——	——
Awake most of the time	——	——	——
SAFETY			
ID bracelet on	2330 AF 0200 AF	0800 JM 1200 JM 1500 JM	1600 HM 2100 HM
Call bell in reach	2330 AF 0200 AF	0800 JM 1200 JM 1500 JM	1600 HM 2100 HM
Side rails up	2330 AF 0200 AF	0800 JM 1200 JM 1500 JM	1600 HM 2100 HM

Don't leave space blank. Write "none" or "N/A," or draw a line through the space.

Flow sheets encourage you to chart care promptly.

to document information. Flow sheets allow you to easily follow trends or changes in the patient's condition.

Teaching sheets

Teaching sheets are used to document patient education and to provide you with information about:
- what the patient needs to learn *(learning needs)*
- the patient's level of understanding after teaching *(evaluation)*
- what was taught *(teaching content)*
- teaching techniques (such as demonstration, role playing, or lecture)
- teaching materials (such as written material or videos).

Forms and more forms

There are several forms for documenting a patient-teaching plan. Many of them incorporate the nursing process as it applies to patient education. (See *Patient-teaching flow sheets.*)

Good morning, class

Because patient education will be an important part of the care plan for your patient, you should look at the teaching sheets to see what teaching has been done, problems that could hinder patient learning, and the patient's level of understanding.

The teaching sheets will tell you:
- tools and techniques that have been used, such as handouts or videos
- names of family members or other caregivers present for the teaching and their level of understanding
- whether the patient has achieved his learning goals and what methods of evaluation were used.

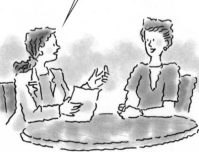

These handouts should help explain your condition.

Discharge summaries

Many facilities combine discharge summaries and patient instructions in one form. This form contains sections for recording patient assessments, patient education, detailed special instructions, and the circumstances of discharge. The form uses a narrative style along with open- and close-ended styles.

One for you, one for your permanent record!

After the discharge summary is complete, one copy of the form is given to the patient and another copy is placed in the medical record. The completed form outlines the patient's care, provides useful information for further teaching and evaluation, and documents that the patient has the information he needs to care for himself or to get further help.

Patient-teaching flow sheets

Here's the first page of a patient-teaching flow sheet. Flow sheets like this one allow all members of the health care team to see at a glance what the patient has learned and what he still needs to learn.

PATIENT-TEACHING FLOW SHEET

ASTHMA

Problems affecting learning

☐ None
☑ Fatigue or pain
☐ Communication problem

☐ Cognitive or sensory impairment
☐ Physical disability

☐ Lack of motivation
Other_____

> This form provides standard learning outcomes for patients with asthma.

LEARNING OUTCOMES	INITIAL TEACHING						REINFORCEMENT					
	Date	Time	Learner	Techniques and tools	Evaluation	Initials	Date	Time	Learner	Techniques and tools	Evaluation	Initials
Basic knowledge												
• Define asthma.	3/9/05	1100	P	E,W	Dv	C B	3/10/05	1100	P	E,W	S	C B
• List two symptoms of asthma.	3/9/05	1100	P	E,W	Dv	C B	3/10/05	1100	P	E,W	S	C B
Medication												
• State the action of theophylline and its effects on the body.	3/9/05	1100	P	E,W	S	C B						
• Name the two inhalers used. Give their onsets, peaks, and durations.	3/9/05	1100	P	E,W,V	Dv	C B						
• Demonstrate the ability to use the inhalers using correct technique.	3/9/05	1100	P	E,W	S	C B						

KEY

Learner
P = patient
S = spouse
M = mother
F = father
D1 = daughter 1_____
D2 = daughter 2_____
S1 = son 1 _____
S2 = son 2 _____
O = other_____

Teaching techniques
D = demonstration
E = explanation
R = role playing

Teaching tools
F = filmstrip
P = physical model
S = slide
V = videotape
W = written material

Evaluation
S = states understanding
D = demonstrates understanding
Dp = demonstrates understanding with physical coaching
Dv = demonstrates understanding with verbal coaching
T = passes written test
N = no indication of learning
NE = not evaluated

Some nice, light reading

Not all facilities use combined forms—some use only narrative discharge summaries. The narrative summary should include:
• the patient's status at admission and discharge
• significant information about the patient's stay in the facility, including resolved and unresolved problems and referrals for continuing care
• instructions given to the patient, members of his family, and other caregivers about medications, treatments, activity, diet, referrals, follow-up appointments, and other special instructions.

The nursing process

One of the most significant advances in nursing has been the development and acceptance of the nursing process. The nursing process is a problem-solving approach to nursing care that offers a structure for applying your knowledge and skills in an organized, goal-oriented manner.

Leave no stone unturned

The cornerstone of clinical nursing, the nursing process provides you with a systematic way to determine your patient's health problems, devise a care plan to address those problems, implement the plan, and evaluate the plan's effectiveness.

When you use the nursing process effectively, it offers you several important advantages:
• Your focus of care is your patient's health problems, not his disease; you promote your patient's participation in his care and encourage independence and compliance—important factors in a positive health outcome.
• Identifying your patient's health problems improves communication by providing you and other nurses with a common list of recognized problems.
• The nursing process provides a consistent, orderly, professional structure; it promotes accountability for nursing activities based on evaluation which, in turn, promotes quality assurance.

Getting started

After you receive your patient assignment, your next step is to gather information about your patient. To do so, you might review the patient's chart the day before clinical or listen to the report from the registered nurse on the morning of clinical.

As you get the report or review the chart, you may find that you begin to cluster assessment findings in your head, identify areas of concern, and start to think of the types of care your patient will need. By doing this, you're starting to apply the nursing process to your patient's care.

Nursing process phases

The nursing process consists of six distinct phases:

 assessment

 nursing diagnosis

 outcome identification

 planning

 implementation

 evaluation. (See *The never-ending process*.)

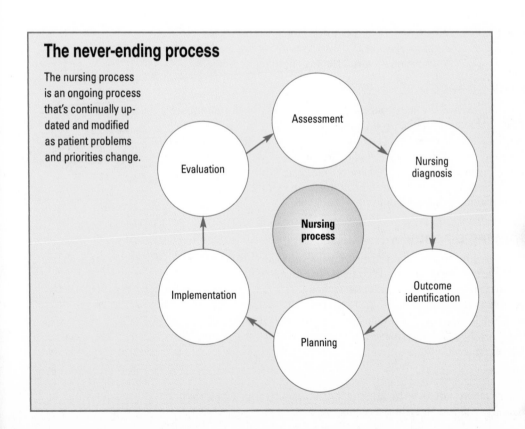

The never-ending process

The nursing process is an ongoing process that's continually updated and modified as patient problems and priorities change.

Assessment

Nursing diagnosis

Evaluation

Nursing process

Outcome identification

Implementation

Planning

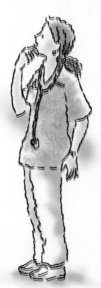

Assessment

Assessment, the first step in the nursing process, begins when you meet your patient. You're already noting such aspects as skin color, speech patterns, and body position. As you move on to perform your formal nursing assessment, you'll collect data in a more structured manner through a nursing history, physical assessment, and review of laboratory and medical information. (See *Establishing priorities for patient assessment.*)

Straight from the patient's mouth

You'll conduct a nursing history to obtain subjective data—that is, information from the patient's point of view. The nursing history provides information on the patient's physical, mental, and emotional functioning. It helps you determine the patient's perception of his health problems and treatments, past coping patterns and their effectiveness, ADLs, preventive health practices, lifestyle, and compliance with medical care. You may obtain this information from other health care professionals, the patient, or his family or caregivers.

Getting physical

You'll collect objective data during the physical examination through inspection, percussion, palpation, and auscultation. You'll then use this information to verify findings in the health history.

From clusters to diagnoses

As you proceed through your patient assessment, you'll probably find yourself starting to group bits of significant data into clusters. You'll use these clusters of assessment findings to formulate nursing diagnoses. For example, a patient's report of shortness of breath while walking short distances coupled with your assessment findings of nasal flaring, rapid respiratory rate, and pursed-lip breathing suggests respiratory problems.

Nursing diagnosis

After clustering the data obtained during your assessment of the patient, your next step is to formulate nursing diagnoses. A nursing diagnosis is a clinical judgment about the patient's response to an actual or potential health problem that a nurse can legally manage. You'll then use this nursing diagnosis to select nursing interventions designed to achieve a certain outcome for which you, the nurse, are accountable.

Good things come in threes

You're now ready to write nursing diagnoses. Make sure that each nursing diagnosis has three components:

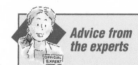

Advice from the experts

Establishing priorities for patient assessment

After completion of an initial assessment, the Joint Commission on Accreditation of Healthcare Organizations requires nurses to use the gathered information in prioritizing their care decisions. To systematically set priorities, follow these steps:
• Identify the patient's problems.
• Identify the patient's risk of injury.
• Identify the patient's need for help with self-care, both in the hospital and after discharge.
• Identify the educational needs of the patient and his family.

   the human response or problem—an actual or potential problem that can be affected by nursing care

   related factors—factors that may precede, contribute to, or be associated with the human response

   signs and symptoms—defining characteristics that lead to the diagnosis.

   For example, a nursing diagnosis for a patient with constipation caused by his use of opioid analgesics for pain might read *Constipation related to use of opioid analgesics as evidenced by passage of hard, formed stools.*

Ah, to eat and breathe

After you've established nursing diagnoses for your patient, you must prioritize them into high-, intermediate-, and low-priority diagnoses. You'll begin your care plan with the highest-priority diagnoses. Maslow's hierarchy of needs can help you set priorities in your care plan. Physiologic needs, the base of Maslow's hierarchy, have the highest priority and include such basic needs as oxygen and food. (See *Maslow's pyramid.*)

Maslow's pyramid

To formulate nursing diagnoses, you must know your patient's needs and values. Of course, physiologic needs—represented by the base of the pyramid in the diagram below—must be met first.

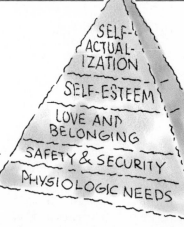

Self-actualization
Recognition and realization of one's potential, growth, health, and autonomy

Self-esteem
Sense of self-worth, self-respect, independence, dignity, privacy, self-reliance

Love and belonging
Affiliation, affection, intimacy, support, reassurance

Safety and security
Safety from physiologic and psychological threat, protection, continuity, stability, lack of danger

Physiologic needs
Oxygen, food, elimination, temperature control, sex, movement, rest, comfort

Outcome identification

The focus of your nursing care is to help your patient reach his highest possible level of independent functioning with minimal risk. If he can't recover completely, the focus of your care is to help him cope physically and emotionally with his impaired or declining health.

Right on target

You should identify realistic, measurable, expected outcomes with reasonable target dates for your patient. *Expected outcomes* are goals the patient should reach as a result of nursing interventions you've planned. (See *Writing excellent outcome statements.*)

Your outcome statement should consist of four parts:

 the specific behavior that shows the patient has reached his goal

criteria for measuring that behavior

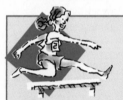

Overcoming obstacles

Writing excellent outcome statements

Does this student's question ring a bell? If so, learn from words of wisdom.

Question

I don't know the first thing about writing outcome statements. What do I need to include?

Words of wisdom

These tips will help you write clear, precise outcome statements:

• When writing expected outcomes in your care plan, always start with a specific action verb that focuses on your patient's behavior. By telling your reader how your patient should *look, walk, eat, drink, turn, cough, speak,* or *stand,* for example, you give a clear picture of how to evaluate progress.

• Avoid starting expected outcome statements with *allow, let, enable,* or similar verbs. Such words focus attention on your own and other health care team members' behavior—not the patient's.

• With many documentation formats, you won't need to include the phrase *The patient will...* with each expected outcome statement. However, you'll have to specify to which person the goals refer when family, friends, or others are directly involved.

Components of an outcome statement

An outcome statement consists of four elements: behavior, measure, condition, and time.

 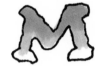 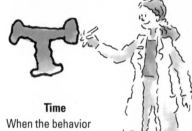

Behavior	**Measure**	**Condition**	**Time**
A desired behavior for the patient; must be observable	Criteria for measuring the behavior; should specify how much, how long, how far, and so on	The conditions under which the behavior should occur	When the behavior should occur

As indicated, the two outcome statements below have these four components.

Ambulate	one flight of stairs	unassisted	by 02/12/05
Demonstrate	measuring radial pulse	before exercising	by 02/12/05

the conditions under which the behavior should occur

when the behavior should occur. (See *Components of an outcome statement*.)

Planning

Now you're ready for the next stage of the nursing process—planning. The nursing care plan is a written plan of action designed to help you deliver quality patient care. The care plan is based on the problems identified during the patient's admission interview. The plan consists of:
• nursing diagnoses
• expected outcomes
• nursing interventions.

Permanent but flexible

The care plan becomes a permanent part of the patient's record and is used by all members of the nursing team. Remember, a patient's problems and needs change, so review the care plan often, and modify it if necessary.

Be sure to include these three steps when writing a care plan:

- prioritizing nursing diagnoses

- selecting appropriate nursing interventions to achieve expected outcomes

- documenting nursing diagnoses, expected outcomes, nursing interventions, and evaluations.

Implementation

Now you're ready to select and implement nursing interventions. Nursing interventions are actions that you and your patient agree will help him reach expected outcomes. Base these interventions on the second part of your nursing diagnosis, the *related factors*.

For example, with a nursing diagnosis of *Impaired physical mobility related to arthritic morning stiffness*, select interventions that reduce or eliminate the patient's stiffness such as mild stretching exercises.

If at first you don't succeed...

How do you come up with interventions? First, consider interventions that you or your patient have successfully tried before. You can also choose interventions from standardized care plans or nursing care plan books, or you can check nursing journals and textbooks for ideas. If these methods don't work, try brainstorming with other nurses and students and asking them about interventions they've used successfully.

Make sure that the interventions you choose are specific and clearly state the necessary action. Note how and when to perform the intervention and include special instructions. *Promote comfort* doesn't tell you what specific action to take, but *Administer ordered analgesic 30 minutes before dressing change* tells you exactly what to do and when to do it.

One size doesn't fit all

Make sure that the interventions you choose fit the patient. Consider the patient's age, condition, developmental level, environment, and values. For instance, if he's a vegetarian, don't write an intervention that requires him to eat lean meat to gain extra protein for healing.

Evaluation

Evaluation is an ongoing process that takes place each time you see your patient. It includes reassessing your patient, comparing

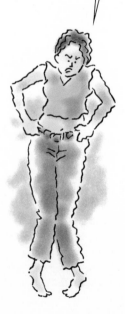

Remember to tailor your care to your patient. When it comes to nursing interventions, one size doesn't fit all!

the findings with the outcome criteria, determining the extent of outcome achievement (whether the outcome was met, partially met, or not met), writing evaluation statements, and revising the care plan. (See *Effective evaluation statements.*)

After evaluating the outcome, be sure to record it in the patient's chart with clear statements that demonstrate his progress toward meeting the expected outcomes.

Nursing care plans

The nursing care plan is a vital source of information about the patient's problems, needs, and goals. It contains detailed instructions for achieving the goals established for the patient and is used to direct care. (See *Tips for top-notch care plans.*)

Your clinical instructor may require you to purchase a certain nursing care plan book. If not, you may want to consider buying

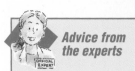

Effective evaluation statements

These evaluation statements clearly describe common outcomes. Note that they include specific details of the care provided and objective evidence of the patient's response to care.

• *Able to describe the signs and symptoms of hyperglycemia* (response to patient education)

• *States leg pain decreased from 9 to 6 (on a scale of 0 to 10) 30 minutes after receiving I.M. meperidine* (response to pain medication within 1 hour of administration)

• *Able to ambulate to chair with a steady gait, approximately 10' unassisted* (tolerance of change or increase in activity)

• *Unable to tolerate removal of O_2, became dyspneic on room air even at rest* (tolerance of treatments)

Tips for top-notch care plans

Use either a traditional or standardized method for recording your care plan. A *traditional care plan* is written from scratch for each patient. A *standardized care plan* saves time because it's predetermined, based on the patient's diagnosis.

No matter which method you use, follow these tips to write an accurate and useful plan:
• Write in ink and sign your name.
• Use clear, concise language, not vague terms or generalities.
• Use standard abbreviations to avoid confusion.
• Review all your assessment data *before* selecting an approach for each problem; if you can't complete the initial assessment, immediately write *insufficient information* on your records.
• Write an expected outcome and a target date for each problem you identify.

• Set realistic initial goals.
• When writing nursing interventions, consider what to watch for and how often, what nursing measures to take and how to perform them, and what to teach the patient and his family before discharge.
• Make each nursing intervention specific.
• Make sure that your interventions match the staff's resources and capabilities.
• Be creative; include a drawing or an innovative procedure if this makes your directions more specific.
• Record all of the patient's problems and concerns so they won't be forgotten.
• Make sure that your plan is implemented correctly.
• Evaluate the results of your plan and discontinue nursing diagnoses that have been resolved; select new approaches, if necessary, for problems that haven't been resolved.

one to help you with care plan development. Be sure to look over each book before selecting one. Different authors emphasize different aspects of the nursing care plan. In the early part of your nursing education, for example, a book that provides in-depth rationales for nursing interventions may be helpful; however, more experienced students may only need a quick list of nursing actions with minimal rationales.

Your patient's nursing care plan may be in one of two styles, *traditional* or *standardized*.

Traditional care plan

The traditional care plan is written from scratch for each patient. Most have three main columns:

 nursing diagnoses

 expected outcomes

 interventions.

Documenting marathon

There may be other columns for the date when the care plan was initiated, target dates for expected outcomes, and the dates for review, revisions, and resolutions. Most forms also have a place for you to sign or initial whenever you make an entry or revision. Although this type of care plan allows you to individualize the care of each patient, it requires lengthy documentation.

Standardized care plan

More commonly, your patient will have a *standardized care plan* that's preprinted to save documentation time. Some standardized plans are classified by medical diagnosis; others, by nursing diagnosis.

Individualizing care plans

Even though these care plans are standardized, they allow you to individualize the plan for each of your patients by adding:
• *"related to" (R/T) statements and signs and symptoms for a nursing diagnosis.* If the form provides a root diagnosis—such as "Pain R/T _____"—you might fill in, "inflammation, as exhibited by grimacing and expressions of pain."
• *time limits for the outcomes to a root statement of the goal.* For example, to the statement, "Perform postural drainage with-

out assistance," you might add, "for 15 minutes immediately upon awakening on the morning of 11/12."
• *frequency of interventions.* To an intervention such as "Perform passive ROM exercises," you might add "twice daily: 1x each morning and evening."
• *specific instructions for interventions.* For the standard intervention, "Elevate patient's head," you might specify, "before sleep, on three pillows." (See *Why stand on tradition? Use a standardized plan.*)

Why stand on tradition? Use a standardized plan

The standardized care plan below is for a patient with a nursing diagnosis of *Impaired tissue integrity.* To customize it to your patient, complete the diagnosis—including signs and symptoms—and fill in the expected outcomes.

> There's a lot less writing with standardized plans.

Date _2/15/05_

Nursing diagnosis
Impaired tissue integrity related to arterial insufficiency

Target date _2/17/05_

Expected outcomes
Attains relief from immediate symptoms: *pain, ulcers, edema*
Voices intent to change aggravating behavior: *will stop smoking immediately*
Maintains collateral circulation: *palpable peripheral pulses, extremities warm and pink with good capillary refill*
Voices intent to follow specific management routines after discharge: *foot care guidelines, exercise regimen as specified by physical therapy department*

Date _2/15/05_

Interventions
• Provide foot care. Administer and monitor treatments according to facility protocols.
• Encourage adherence to an exercise regimen as tolerated.
• Educate the patient about risk factors and prevention of injury. Refer the patient to a stop-smoking program.
• Maintain adequate hydration. Monitor I/O _q8h._
• To increase arterial blood supply to the extremities, elevate head of bed _6" to 8"._
• Additional interventions: *inspect skin integrity q8h.*

Date _____

Outcomes evaluation
Attained relief of immediate symptoms: _____
Voiced intent to change aggravating behavior: _____
Maintained collateral circulation: _____
Voiced intent to follow specific management routines after discharge: _____

Critical pathways

Critical pathways are standardized care plans used by interdisciplinary teams, not just nurses. They include assessment criteria, interventions, treatments, and outcomes for specific conditions according to a time line.

Complete coverage

Think of the pathway as a predetermined checklist describing the tasks you and the patient must accomplish. Unlike a nursing care plan, its focus is multidisciplinary, covering all of the patient's problems, not just those identified during a nursing assessment. (See *Take the critical pathway.*)

Critical pathways cover the key events that must occur before the patient's target discharge date. These events include:
- consultations
- diagnostic tests
- treatments
- medications
- procedures
- activities
- diet
- patient teaching
- discharge planning
- achievement of anticipated outcomes.

Concept mapping

Your clinical instructor may ask you to use concept mapping to show the flow of your critical thinking during patient care. Concept mapping allows your clinical instructor to see whether you understand the relationship between important concepts required to provide skillful care for your patient.

A big advantage of concept mapping over nursing care plans is that it requires much less writing time — something all nursing students need! Concept mapping also allows you to be creative and individualize patient care.

Developing a concept map

When developing a concept map, don't be too concerned about putting ideas in the "wrong" places. It's more important to write the idea down. When you worry about writing ideas in proper places, you revert back to linear, rather than critical, thinking.

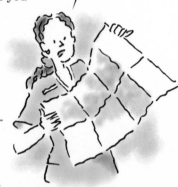

Don't let concept maps intimidate you! Remember that writing down the information is more important than where you put it.

Take the critical pathway

At any point in a treatment course, a glance at the critical pathway allows you to compare the patient's progress and your performance as a caregiver with standards. The standard critical pathway below outlines care for a patient with a colon resection.

CRITICAL PATHWAY: COLON RESECTION WITHOUT COLOSTOMY				
	Patient visit	**Presurgery day 1**	**Day 0 O.R. day**	**Postoperative day 1**
Assessments	History and physical with breast, rectal, and pelvic examinations Nursing assessment	Nursing admission assessment	Nursing admission assessment on TBA patients in holding area Postoperative review of systems assessment*	Review of systems assessment*
Consults	Social service consult Physical therapy consult	Notify referring doctor of impending admission		
Labs and diagnostics	Complete blood count (CBC) PT/PTT Electrocardiogram Chest X-ray (CXR) Chemistry profile CT scan ABD w/wo contrast CT scan pelvis Urinalysis Barium enema and flexible sigmoidoscopy or colonoscopy Biopsy report	Type and screen for patients with Hg level < 10	Type and screen for patients in holding area with Hg level < 10	CB
Interventions	Many or all of the above labs and diagnostics will have already been done. Check all results and fax to the surgeon's	Admit by 0800 Check for bowel preparation orders Bowel preparation* Antiembolism stockings Incentive spirometry Ankle exercises* I.V. access* Routine VS* Pneumatic inflation boots	Shave and prepare in operating room NG tube maintenance* I/O VS per routine* Foley care* Incentive spirometry* Ankle exercises* I.V. site care* HOB 30° Safety measures* Wound care* Mouth care*	NG tube maintenance* I/O* VS per routine* Foley care* Incentive spirometry* Ankle exercises* I.V. site care* HOB 30°* Safety measures* Wound care* Mouth care* Antiembolism stockings
I.V.s		I.V. fluids, $D_5\frac{1}{2}$ NSS	I.V. fluids, D_5LR	I.V. fluids, D_5LR
Medication	Prescribe GoLYTELY or NuLYTELY 1000-1400 Neomycin @ 1400, 1500, and 2200 Erythromycin @ 1400, 1500, and 2200	GoLYTELY or NuLYTELY 1000-1400 Erythromycin @ 1400, 1500, and 2200 Neomycin @ 1400, 1500, and 2200	Preoperative ABX in holding area Postoperative ABX × 2 doses PCA (basal rate 0.5 mg) subQ heparin	
Diet/GI	Clears presurgery day NPO after midnight	Clears presurgery day NPO after midnight	NPO/NG tube	
Activity			4 hours after surgery ambulate with abdominal binder* D/C pneumatic inflation boots after patient ambulates	Ambulate t.i.d. with abdominal binder* May shower Physical therapy b.i.d.

The pathway designates a specific time frame for patient care activities.

The pathway is organized into categories based on the patient's medical diagnosis.

The pathway lists tasks that the patient and caregivers need to accomplish.

| KEY: *= NSG Activities
V = Variance
N = No Var. | 1.   2.   3.
V̶   V̶   V̶
Ⓝ   N   N | 1.   2.   3.
V̶   V̶   V̶
Ⓝ   Ⓝ   Ⓝ | 1.   2.   3.
V̶   V̶   V̶
Ⓝ   Ⓝ   Ⓝ | 1.   2.   3.
V̶   V̶   V̶
Ⓝ   Ⓝ   Ⓝ |
| **Signatures:** | 1. C. Molloy, RN
2.
3. | 1. M Connel, RN
2. J. Smith, RN
3. P. Joseph, RN | 1. L. Singer, RN
2. J. Smith, RN
3. P. Joseph, RN | 1. L. Singer, RN
2. J. Smith, RN
3. P. Joseph, RN |

(continued)

Take the critical pathway *(continued)*

CRITICAL PATHWAY: COLON RESECTION WITHOUT COLOSTOMY

	Postoperative day 2	Postoperative day 3	Postoperative day 4	Postoperative day 5
Assessments	Review of systems assessment*	Review of systems assessment*	Review of systems assessment	Review of systems assessment*
Consults		Dietary consult		Oncology consult if indicated (Dukes B2 or C or high-risk lesion) (or to be done as outpatient)
Labs and diagnostics	Electrolyte 7 (EL-7) CXR	CBC EL-7	Pathology results on chart	CBC EL-7
Interventions	Discontinue NG tube if possible* (per guidelines) I/O* VS per routine* Discontinue Foley* Ambulating* Incentive spirometry* Ankle exercises* I.V. site care* HOB 30°* Safety measures* Wound care* Mouth care* Antiembolism stockings	I/O* VS per routine* Incentive spirometry* Ankle exercises* I.V. site care* Safety measures* Wound care* Antiembolism stockings	I/O* VS per routine* Incentive spirometry* Ankle exercises* I.V. site care* Safety measures* Wound care* Antiembolism stockings	Consider staple removal Replace with Steri-Strips Assess that patient has met discharge criteria* Discontinue saline lock
I.V.s	I.V. fluids $D_5\frac{1}{2}$ NSS+ MVI	I.V. convert to saline lock	Continue saline lock	Disco...
Medication	PCA (0.5 mg basal rate)	Discontinue PCA P.O. analgesia Resume routine home meds	P.O. analgesia Preoperative meds	P.O. analgesia Preoperative meds
Diet/GI	Discontinue NG tube per guidelines: (Clamp tube at 8 a.m. if no N/V and residual < 200 ml, D/C tube @ 1200)* (Check with doctor first)	Clears if+bm/flatus Advance to postoperative diet if tolerating clears (at least one tray of clears)	House	House
Activity	Ambulate q.i.d. with abdominal binder* May shower Physical therapy b.i.d.	Ambulate at least q.i.d. with abdominal binder* May shower Physical therapy b.i.d.	Ambulate at least q.i.d. with abdominal binder* May shower Physical therapy b.i.d.	
Teaching	Reinforce preoperative teaching* Patient and family education p.r.n.* Re: family screening	Reinforce preoperative teaching* Patient and family education p.r.n.* Re: family screening Begin discharge teaching	Reinforce preoperative teaching* Patient and family education p.r.n.* Discharge teaching re: reportable s/s, follow-up, and wound care*	Review all discharge instructions and Rx including:* follow-up appointments: with surgeon within 3 weeks with oncologist within 1 month if indicated
KEY: * = NSG Activities **V** = Variance **N** = No Var.	1. 2. 3. V V V Ⓝ Ⓝ Ⓝ	1. 2. 3. V V V Ⓝ Ⓝ Ⓝ	1. 2. 3. V V V Ⓝ Ⓝ Ⓝ	1. 2. 3. V V V Ⓝ Ⓝ N
Signatures:	1. _A. McCarthy, RN_ 2. _R. Moyer, RN_ 3. _L. Waters, RN_	1. _A. McCarthy, RN_ 2. _R. Moyer, RN_ 3. _L. Waters, RN_	1. _L. Singer, RN_ 2. _J. Smith, RN_ 3. _P. Joseph, RN_	1. _L. Singer, RN_ 2. _J. Smith, RN_ 3.

> The pathway lists key events that must occur before the patient's discharge date.

A fresh start

To develop a concept map, start with a clean sheet of paper. Some students prefer unlined paper and colored pencils or pens to promote creative thinking. Then follow these steps:

After you've assessed your patient, place a box representing the patient in the middle of your paper. In this box, write the patient's medical diagnosis or chief complaint. Be brief! By placing the patient in the center of the page, your focus is clearly patient-centered.

Write the major problems or nursing diagnoses in boxes surrounding the patient with the pertinent supporting data.

Use lines to connect the patient to the nursing diagnoses. Lines may also be drawn between related nursing diagnoses. For example, for a postoperative patient experiencing constipation caused by use of opioid analgesics, you would draw a line between the nursing diagnoses of "Acute pain" and "Constipation" to show that you understand that they're related.

Prioritize each nursing diagnosis by numbering the boxes.

Write expected outcomes for each nursing diagnosis; place each outcome in its own box because corresponding interventions will be different for each outcome. Connect these boxes by lines to the appropriate nursing diagnoses.

In the same manner, write interventions in a box for each outcome, followed by evaluations. Draw lines between each part of the nursing process to show concepts that are related.

A job well done!

Your concept map is complete — for now. You'll need to continually update it throughout the clinical day.

Using a concept map

Use the concept map during your clinical day to guide your patient care. Carry it in your pocket or on your clipboard so you can refer to it often. Keeping it to one page will make it easier to use. Make notes directly on the concept map to update and revise it as necessary.

Your instructor may have you take out the concept map to discuss patient care concepts. For example, you can use the concept map to explain the relationships between incentive spirometry and respiratory assessment findings in your postoperative patient. The concept map allows you to see relationships more clearly at a glance.

Interdisciplinary team

There's no "I" in TEAM. But there's a dietitian, a social worker, an occupational therapist...

Nurses aren't the only health care professionals involved in patient care. You'll need to collaborate with an interdisciplinary team to meet the diverse needs of your patients.

Share and share alike

The focus of an interdisciplinary team is on the patient and patient outcomes. Each team member shares responsibility for achieving these outcomes. To provide more effective and comprehensive care, you need to understand each team member's role.

Members of the health care team include the:
• *registered dietitian*, who assesses and monitors nutritional needs, makes nutritional recommendations, and provides patient education
• *social worker*, who provides support and counseling to patients and their families and helps with financial difficulties
• *occupational therapist*, who assists the patient in performing ADLs, participating in recreation, and working to his highest functional level
• *physical therapist*, who provides therapy to improve or restore physical functioning and prevent deconditioning
• *respiratory therapist*, who monitors and provides airway management
• *pastoral care specialist*, who provides spiritual and religious support to patients and their families
• *pharmacist*, who reviews, prepares, and dispenses the patient's medications; provides information and guidance in the preparation and administration of medications; and provides patient education.

Passing notes is permitted!

When you're reviewing the patient's chart, be sure to read the progress notes written by other members of the health care team. These notes will provide you with important information about your patient.

If you have questions about the patient's condition or treatment, contact the appropriate team members for more information. For example, the pharmacist can provide information about how to space medications to eliminate drug or food interactions, whereas the physical therapist can provide guidelines on how to safely transfer a patient with fractures from the bed to a chair.

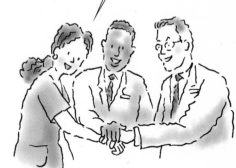

Together, let's provide great patient care!

Play well with others

You'll also need to coordinate care with other team members. For example, medicating your postoperative patient before respiratory exercises helps the patient cough and deep-breathe more effectively with the respiratory therapist. When working with the other team members, remember to use good communication skills. Above all, treat all team members with respect, and they'll respect you in turn!

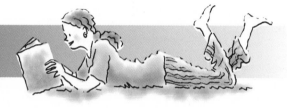

Take a break!

Mapping out the concept map

Follow these steps and use the case study to create a concept map. Answers are on the next page.

Case study

Mr. Jones, a 58-year-old male, was admitted to the medical-surgical floor with cholecystitis. The patient complains of pain in his epigastric area, nausea, and vomiting. His vital signs are: heart rate 102 beats/minute, blood pressure 142/88 mm Hg, oral temperature 100.4° F, and respiration 18 breaths/minute.

The patient rates the pain an 8 on the numeric scale of 0 to 10. (10 is the most extreme degree of pain, and 0 is the absence of pain.) A nasogastric (NG) tube has been placed and is connected to low, intermittent wall suction and an I.V. of $D_5 1/2$ NSS has been started at 75 ml/hr. Mr. Jones is scheduled for a laparoscopic cholecystectomy the next day.

Steps

1. Assess patient to collect clinical data.

2. Write patient's chief complaint in the middle of a sheet of paper.

3. Write nursing diagnoses in boxes around the reason patient is seeking health care.

4. Categorize assessment data under appropriate nursing diagnosis.

5. Analyze relationship among nursing diagnoses and draw lines to indicate this relationship.

6. On another piece of paper, identify patient goals, outcomes, and nursing interventions for each nursing diagnosis on the concept map. Instead of using another piece of paper, you may wish to create additional boxes that include the goals, outcomes, and interventions and link these boxes to the related nursing diagnoses.

Answer key

This concept map is one example of many possibilities for this patient.

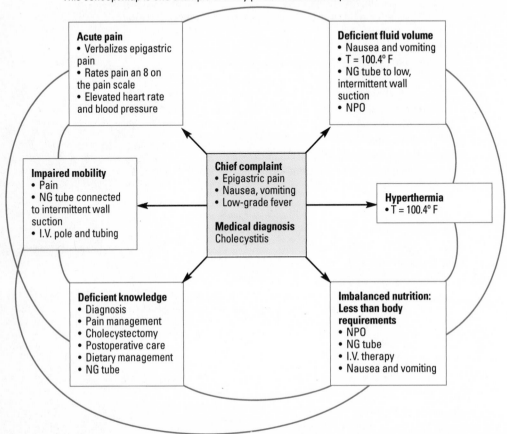

Acute pain
• Verbalizes epigastric pain
• Rates pain an 8 on the pain scale
• Elevated heart rate and blood pressure

Deficient fluid volume
• Nausea and vomiting
• T = 100.4° F
• NG tube to low, intermittent wall suction
• NPO

Impaired mobility
• Pain
• NG tube connected to intermittent wall suction
• I.V. pole and tubing

Chief complaint
• Epigastric pain
• Nausea, vomiting
• Low-grade fever

Medical diagnosis
Cholecystitis

Hyperthermia
• T = 100.4° F

Deficient knowledge
• Diagnosis
• Pain management
• Cholecystectomy
• Postoperative care
• Dietary management
• NG tube

Imbalanced nutrition: Less than body requirements
• NPO
• NG tube
• I.V. therapy
• Nausea and vomiting

The following is an example of a goal, outcomes, and interventions for the nursing diagnosis *Acute pain*. If you didn't follow this approach and added additional boxes containing the goal, outcomes, and interventions and linked these to the nursing diagnoses... you're also correct!

　　Problem: Acute pain
　　Goal: Pain control
　　Outcome: Patient's pain remains below 3 on a 10-point scale

Nursing pain interventions	Evaluation
Assess pain using pain scale.	*This section will include the patient's responses to the interventions on the left.*
Medicate patient for pain, according to the doctor's orders.	
Instruct patient on use of PCA, if appropriate.	
Position patient for comfort.	
Use techniques of relaxation, meditation, or guided imagery.	

Part IV   Preparing for the future

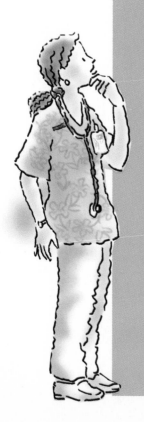

9

Preparing for the NCLEX®

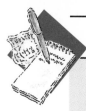

Just the facts

In this chapter, you'll learn:

♦ why you must take the NCLEX®

♦ what you need to know about taking the exam by computer

♦ strategies to use when answering exam questions

♦ how to avoid common mistakes when taking the exam.

NCLEX® basics

Passing the National Council Licensure Examination (NCLEX®) is an important landmark in your career as a nurse. The first step on your way to passing the NCLEX® exam is to understand what it is and how it's administered.

NCLEX® structure

The *NCLEX®* is a test written by nurses who, like most of your nursing instructors, have a master's degree and clinical expertise in a particular area. Only one small difference distinguishes nurses who write NCLEX® questions: They're trained to write questions in a style particular to the NCLEX®.

If you've completed an accredited nursing program, you've already taken numerous tests written by nurses with backgrounds and experiences similar to those of the nurses who write for this exam. The test-taking experience you've already gained will help you pass the exam. So your review should be just that — a review.

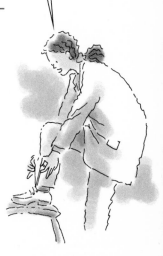

Preparing for your licensing exam is a key step in your nursing career.

What's the point?

The exam is designed for one purpose: namely, to determine whether it's appropriate for you to receive a license to practice as a nurse. By passing the exam, you demonstrate that you possess the minimum level of knowledge necessary to practice nursing safely.

Mix 'em up

In nursing school, you probably took courses organized according to the medical model. Courses were separated into such subjects as medical-surgical, pediatric, maternal-neonatal, and psychiatric nursing. In contrast, the NCLEX® is integrated, meaning that different subjects are mixed together.

As you answer NCLEX® questions, you may encounter patients in any stage of life, from neonatal to geriatric. These patients — *clients*, in NCLEX® lingo — may be of any background, may be completely well or extremely ill, and may have any of a variety of disorders.

Client needs, front and center

The exam draws questions from four categories of client needs that were developed by the National Council of State Boards of Nursing (NCSBN), the organization that sponsors and manages the exam. *Client needs categories* ensure that many topics appear on every examination.

The NCSBN developed client needs categories after conducting a work-study analysis of new nurses. All aspects of nursing care observed in the study were broken down into four categories. Two categories were broken down further into subcategories. (See *Client needs categories*.)

The whole kit and caboodle

The categories and subcategories are used to develop the exam's *test plan*, the content guidelines for the distribution of test questions. Question-writers and the people who put the examination together use the test plan and client needs categories to make sure that a full spectrum of nursing content is covered in the exam. Client needs categories appear in most exam review and question-and-answer books, including this one.

Now you see 'em, now you don't

As a test-taker, you don't have to concern yourself with client needs categories. You'll see these categories for each question and answer in this book, but they'll be invisible on the actual exam.

Client needs categories

Each question on the NCLEX® is assigned a category based on client needs. This chart lists client needs categories and subcategories and the percentages of each type of question that appear on the examination.

Category	Subcategories	Percentage of NCLEX® questions
Safe, effective care environment	• Management of care	13% to 19%
	• Safety and infection control	8% to 14%
Health promotion and maintenance	—	6% to 12%
Psychosocial integrity	—	6% to 12%
Physiological integrity	• Basic care and comfort	6% to 12%
	• Pharmacological and parenteral therapies	13% to 19%
	• Reduction of risk potential	13% to 19%
	• Physiological adaptation	11% to 17%

Testing by computer

Like many standardized tests today, the exam is administered by computer. That means you won't be filling in empty circles, sharpening pencils, or erasing frantically. It also means that you must become familiar with computer tests if you aren't already. Fortunately, the skills required to take the exam on a computer are simple enough to allow you to focus on the questions, not the keyboard.

Q&A

Depending on the question format, when you take the test, you'll be presented with a question and four or more possible answers, a blank space in which to enter your answer, or a figure on which you must click to select the correct area.

Feeling smart? Think hard!

The exam is a *computer-adaptive test,* meaning that the computer reacts to the answers you give, supplying more difficult questions if you answer correctly and slightly easier questions if you answer incorrectly. Each test is thus uniquely adapted to the individual test-taker.

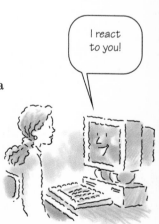

I react to you!

A matter of time

You have a great deal of flexibility with the time you spend on individual questions. The examination lasts a maximum of 6 hours, however, so don't waste time. If you fail to answer a set number of questions within 6 hours, the computer will determine that you lack minimum competency.

Most students have plenty of time to complete the test, so take as much time as you need to get the question right without wasting time. Keep moving at a decent pace to help you maintain concentration.

Difficult items = Good news

If you find as you progress through the test that the questions seem to be increasingly difficult, it's a good sign. The more questions you answer correctly, the more difficult the questions become.

Some students, however, knowing that questions get progressively harder, focus on the degree of difficulty of subsequent questions to try to figure out if they're answering questions correctly. Avoid the temptation to do this, as it may get you off track. Stay focused on selecting the best answer for each question that's put before you.

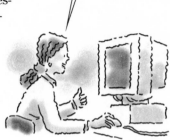

The harder it gets, the better I do.

I'm free!

The computer test finishes when one of the following events occurs:
• You demonstrate minimum competency, according to the computer program.
• You demonstrate a lack of minimum competency, according to the computer program.
• You've answered the maximum number of questions (265 total questions).
• You've used the maximum time allowed (6 hours).

Unlocking the NCLEX® mystery

In 2003, the NCSBN added alternate-format items to the exam. However, most of the questions on the exam are four-option, multiple-choice items with only one correct answer. Regardless of the type, certain strategies can help you understand and answer any question.

Alternate formats

The first type of alternate-format item is the *multiple-response, multiple-choice question*. Unlike a traditional multiple-choice question, each multiple-response, multiple-choice question has more than one correct answer for every question and it may contain more than four possible answer options. You'll recognize this type of question because it will ask you to select *all* answers that apply—not just the *best* answer (as may be requested in the more traditional multiple-choice questions).

All or nothing

Keep in mind that, for each multiple-response, multiple-choice question, you *must select at least two answers* and you *must select all correct answers* for the item to be counted as correct. On the exam, there's no partial credit in scoring these items.

Don't go blank!

The second type of alternate-format item is the *fill-in-the-blank* question. These questions require you to provide the answer yourself, rather than select it from a list of options. There are two kinds of fill-in-the-blank questions. One kind requires you to perform a calculation and type your answer (a number, without any words, commas, or spaces) in the blank space provided after the question. The second kind asks you to prioritize the options and type the correct order of the numbers in the blank space.

Master that mouse!

The final type of alternate-format item is a question that asks you to identify an area on an illustration or graphic. For these so-called "*hot-spot" questions*, the computerized exam will ask you to place your cursor and click over the correct area on an illustration. Try to be as precise as possible when marking the location. As with the fill-in-the-blank questions, the identification questions on the computerized exam may require extremely precise answers for them to be considered correct.

The standard is still the standard

The NCSBN hasn't yet established a percentage of alternate-format items to be administered to each candidate. In fact, your exam may contain only one alternate-format item. So relax; the standard, four-option, multiple-choice format questions make up the bulk of the test. (See *Sample exam questions*, page 186.)

Sample exam questions

Sometimes, getting used to the format is as important as knowing the material. Try your hand at these sample questions and you'll have a leg up when you take the real test!

Sample four-option, multiple-choice question

A client's arterial blood gas (ABG) results are as follows: pH, 7.16; $Paco_2$, 80 mm Hg; Pao_2, 46 mm Hg; HCO_3^-, 24 mEq/L; Sao_2, 81%. This ABG result represents which condition?

1. Metabolic acidosis
2. Metabolic alkalosis
3. Respiratory acidosis
4. Respiratory alkalosis

Correct answer: 3

Sample multiple-response, multiple-choice question

The nurse is caring for a 45-year-old married woman who has undergone hemicolectomy for colon cancer. The woman has two children. Which concepts about families should the nurse keep in mind when providing care for this client? Select all that apply:

1. Illness in one family member can affect all members.
2. Family roles don't change because of illness.
3. A family member may have more than one role at a time in the family.
4. Children typically aren't affected by adult illness.
5. The effects of an illness on a family depend on the stage of the family's life cycle.
6. Changes in sleeping and eating patterns may be signs of stress in a family.

Correct answer: 1, 3, 5, 6

Sample "hot-spot" question

An elderly client has a history of aortic stenosis. Identify the area where the nurse should place the stethoscope to best hear the murmur.

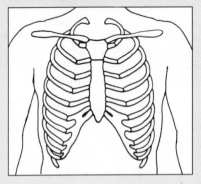

Correct answer:

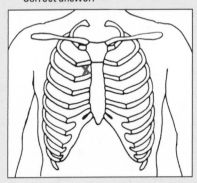

Sample fill-in-the blank calculation question

An infant who weighs 8 kg is to receive ampicillin (Omnipen) 25 mg/kg I.V. every 6 hours. How many milligrams should the nurse administer per dose?

—————

Correct answer: 200

Sample fill-in-the blank prioritizing question

When teaching an antepartal client about the passage of the fetus through the birth canal during labor, the nurse describes the cardinal mechanisms of labor. Place these events in the sequence in which they occur:

1. Flexion
2. External rotation
3. Descent
4. Expulsion
5. Internal rotation
6. Extension

—————

Correct answer: 315624

Understanding the question

Exam questions are commonly lengthy. As a result, it's easy to become overloaded with information. To focus on the question and avoid becoming overwhelmed, apply proven strategies for answering the questions, including:
- determining what the question is asking
- determining relevant facts about the client
- rephrasing the question in your mind
- choosing the best option(s) or answer to enter.

Determine what the question is asking

Read the question twice. If the answer isn't apparent, rephrase the question in simpler, more personal terms. Breaking down the question into easier, less intimidating terms may help you focus more accurately on the correct answer.

Give it a try

For example, a question might be, "A 74-year-old client with a history of heart failure is admitted to the coronary care unit with pulmonary edema. He's intubated and placed on a mechanical ventilator. Which parameter should the nurse monitor closely to assess the client's response to a bolus dose of furosemide (Lasix) I.V.?"

The options for this question — numbered from 1 to 4 — might be:
1. Daily weight
2. 24-hour intake and output
3. Serum sodium levels
4. Hourly urine output

Hocus, focus on the question

Read the question again, ignoring all details except what's being asked. Focus on the last line of the question. It asks you to select the appropriate assessment for monitoring a client who received a bolus of furosemide I.V.

Determine what facts about the client are relevant

Next, sort out the relevant client information. Start by asking whether any of the information provided about the client isn't relevant. For instance, do you need to know that the client has been admitted to the coronary care unit? Probably not; his reaction to I.V. furosemide won't be affected by his location in the hospital.

Determine what you do know about the client. In the example, you know that:
- he just received an I.V. bolus of furosemide, a crucial fact

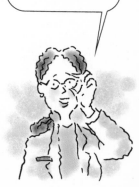

Focusing on what the question is really asking can help you choose the correct answer.

• he has pulmonary edema, the most fundamental aspect of the client's underlying condition
• he's intubated and placed on a mechanical ventilator, suggesting that his pulmonary edema is serious
• he's 74 years old and has a history of heart failure, a fact that may or may not be relevant.

Rephrase the question

After you've determined relevant information about the client and the question being asked, consider rephrasing the question to make it more clear. Eliminate jargon and put the question in simpler, more personal terms. Here's how you might rephrase the question in the example: "My client has pulmonary edema. He requires intubation and mechanical ventilation. He's 74 years old and has a history of heart failure. He received an I.V. bolus of furosemide. What assessment parameter should I monitor?"

Choose the best option

Armed with all the information you now have, it's time to select an option. You know that the client received an I.V. bolus of furosemide, a diuretic. You know that monitoring fluid intake and output is a key nursing intervention for a client taking a diuretic, a fact that eliminates options 1 and 3 (daily weight and serum sodium levels), narrowing the answer down to option 2 or 4 (24-hour intake and output or hourly urine output).

Can I use a lifeline?

You also know that the drug was administered by I.V. bolus, suggesting a rapid effect. (In fact, furosemide administered by I.V. bolus takes effect almost immediately.) Monitoring the client's 24-hour intake and output would be appropriate for assessing the effects of repeated doses of furosemide. Hourly urine output, however, is most appropriate in this situation because it monitors the immediate effect of this rapid-acting drug.

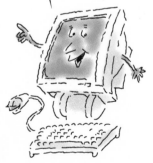

I can be ambivalent. More than one answer may be correct. But there's always a "best" answer!

Key strategies

Regardless of the type of question, four key strategies will help you determine the correct answer for each question. (See *Strategies for success*.) These strategies are:
• considering the nursing process
• referring to Maslow's hierarchy of needs
• reviewing patient safety
• reflecting on principles of therapeutic communication.

Advice from the experts

Strategies for success

Keeping a few main strategies in mind as you answer each exam question can help ensure greater success. These four strategies are critical for answering exam questions correctly:
• If the question asks what you should do in a situation, use the nursing process to determine which step in the process would be next.

• If the question asks what the client needs, use Maslow's hierarchy to determine which need to address first.
• If the question indicates that the client doesn't have an urgent physiologic need, focus on the patient's safety.
• If the question involves communicating with a patient, use the principles of therapeutic communication.

Nursing process

One of the ways to answer a question is to apply the nursing process. Steps in the nursing process include:
• assessment
• analysis
• planning
• implementation
• evaluation.

First things first

The nursing process may provide insights that help you analyze a question. According to the nursing process, assessment comes before analysis, which comes before planning, which comes before implementation, which comes before evaluation.

You're halfway to the correct answer when you encounter a four-option, multiple-choice question that asks you to assess the situation and then provides two assessment options and two implementation options. You can immediately eliminate the implementation options, which then gives you, at worst, a 50-50 chance of selecting the correct answer. Use this sample question to apply the nursing process:

A client returns from an endoscopic procedure during which he was sedated. Before offering the client food, which action should the nurse take?
1. Assess the client's respiratory status.
2. Check the client's gag reflex.
3. Place the client in a side-lying position.
4. Have the client drink a few sips of water.

Assess before intervening

According to the nursing process, the nurse must assess a client before performing an intervention. Does the question indicate that the client has been properly assessed? No, it doesn't. Therefore, you can eliminate options 3 and 4 because they're both interventions.

That leaves options 1 and 2, both of which are assessments. Your nursing knowledge should tell you the correct answer — in this case, option 2. The sedation required for an endoscopic procedure may impair the client's gag reflex, so you would assess the gag reflex before giving food to the client to reduce the risk of aspiration and airway obstruction.

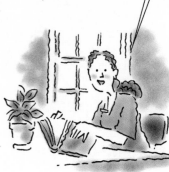

Say it 1,000 times: Studying is fun... studying is fun... studying is fun...

Final elimination

Why not select option 1, assessing the client's respiratory status? You might select this option, but the question is specifically asking about offering the client food, an action that wouldn't be taken if the client's respiratory status was at all compromised. In this case, you're making a judgment based on the phrase, "Before offering the client food." If the question was trying to test your knowledge of respiratory depression following an endoscopic procedure, it probably wouldn't mention a function — such as giving food to a client — that clearly occurs only after the client's respiratory status has been stabilized.

Maslow's hierarchy

Knowledge of Maslow's hierarchy of needs can be a vital tool for establishing priorities on the examination. Maslow's theory states that physiologic needs are the most basic human needs of all. Only after physiologic needs have been met can safety concerns be addressed. Only after safety concerns are met can concerns involving love and belonging be addressed, and so forth. Apply the principles of Maslow's hierarchy of needs to this sample question:

A client complains of severe pain 2 days after surgery. Which action should the nurse perform first?
1. Offer reassurance to the client that he will feel less pain tomorrow.
2. Allow the client time to verbalize his feelings.
3. Check the client's vital signs.
4. Administer an analgesic.

Phys before psych

In this example, two of the options — 3 and 4 — address physiologic needs. Options 1 and 2 address psychosocial concerns. According to Maslow, physiologic needs must be met before psychosocial needs, so you can eliminate options 1 and 2.

Final elimination

Now, use your nursing knowledge to choose the best answer from the two remaining options. In this case, option 3 is correct because the client's vital signs should be checked before administering an analgesic (assessment before intervention). When prioritizing according to Maslow's hierarchy, remember your ABCs—airway, breathing, circulation—to help you further prioritize. Check for a patent airway before addressing breathing. Check breathing before checking the health of the cardiovascular system.

One caveat...

Just because an option appears on the exam doesn't mean it's a viable choice for the client referred to in the question. Always examine your choice in light of your knowledge and experience. Ask yourself, "Does this choice make sense for this client?" Allow yourself to eliminate choices—even ones that might normally take priority—if they don't make sense for a particular client's situation.

Patient safety

As you might expect, patient safety takes high priority on the exam. You'll encounter many questions that can be answered by asking yourself, "Which answer will best ensure the safety of this client?" Use patient safety criteria for situations involving laboratory values, drug administration, or nursing care procedures.

Client 1st, equipment 2nd

You may encounter a question in which some options address the client and others address the equipment. When in doubt, select an option relating to the client; never place equipment before a client.

For instance, suppose a question asks what the nurse should do first when entering a client's room where an infusion pump alarm is sounding. If two options deal with the infusion pump, one with the infusion tubing, and another with the client's catheter insertion site, select the one relating to the client's catheter insertion site. Always check the client first; the equipment can wait.

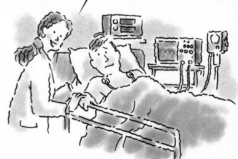

Patient safety takes a high priority on the exam.

Therapeutic communication

Some exam questions focus on the nurse's ability to communicate effectively with the client. Therapeutic communication incorporates verbal or nonverbal responses and involves:
• listening to the client
• understanding the client's needs
• promoting clarification and insight about the client's condition.

Room for improvement

Like other exam questions, those dealing with therapeutic communication require choosing the best response. First, eliminate options that indicate the use of poor therapeutic communication techniques, such as those in which the nurse:
• tells the client what to do without regard to the client's feelings or desires (the "do this" response)
• asks a question that can be answered "yes" or "no," or with another one-syllable response
• seeks reasons for the client's behavior
• implies disapproval of the client's behavior
• offers false reassurances
• attempts to interpret the client's behavior rather than allowing the client to verbalize his own feelings
• offers a response that focuses on the nurse, not the client.

Ah, that's better!

When answering exam questions, look for responses that:
• allow the client time to think and reflect
• encourage the client to talk
• encourage the client to describe a particular experience
• reflect that the nurse has listened to the client such as through paraphrasing the client's response.

Avoiding pitfalls

Even the most knowledgeable students can get tripped up on certain exam questions. (See *A tricky question*.) Students commonly cite three areas that can be difficult for unwary test-takers:

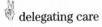 knowing the difference between the NCLEX® and the "real world"

 delegating care

 knowing laboratory values.

Advice from the experts

A tricky question

The exam occasionally asks a particular kind of question called the "further teaching" question, which involves patient-teaching situations. These questions can be tricky. You'll have to choose the response that suggests that the patient hasn't learned the correct information. Here's an example:

37. A client undergoes a total hip replacement. Which statement by the client indicates that she requires further teaching?

1. "I'll need to keep several pillows between my legs at night."
2. "I'll need to remember not to cross my legs. It's such a bad habit."
3. "The occupational therapist is showing me how to use a 'sock puller' to help me get dressed."
4. "I don't know if I'll be able to get off that low toilet seat at home by myself."

The answer you should choose here is option 4 because it indicates that the client has a poor understanding of the precautions required after a total hip replacement and that she needs further teaching. Remember: If you see the phrase further teaching or further instruction, you're looking for a wrong answer by the patient.

NCLEX® versus the real world

Some students who take the exam have extensive practical experience in health care. For example, many test-takers have worked as licensed practical nurses or nursing assistants. In one of those capacities, test-takers might have been exposed to less than optimum clinical practice and may carry those experiences over to the exam.

However, the NCLEX® is a textbook examination—not a test of clinical skills. Take the exam with the understanding that what happens in the real world may differ from what the exam and your nursing school say should happen.

Don't take shortcuts

If you've had practical experience in health care, you may know a quicker way to perform a procedure or tricks to get by when you don't have the right equipment. Situations such as staff shortages may force you to improvise. On the exam, such scenarios can lead to trouble. Always check your practical experiences against textbook nursing care, taking care to select the response that follows the textbook.

> Remember, this is an exam, not the real world.

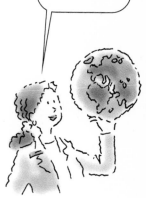

Delegating care

On the exam, you may encounter questions that assess your ability to delegate care. Delegating care involves coordinating the efforts of other health care workers to provide effective care for your client. On the exam, you may be asked to assign duties to:

• licensed practical nurses or licensed vocational nurses
• nursing assistants
• other support staff.

In addition, you'll be asked to decide when to notify a doctor, a social worker, or another hospital staff member. In each case, you'll have to decide when, where, and how to delegate.

Should's and shouldn'ts

As a general rule, it's okay to delegate actions that involve stable clients or standard, unchanging procedures. Bathing, feeding, dressing, and transferring clients are examples of procedures that can be delegated.

Be careful not to delegate complicated or complex activities. In addition, don't delegate activities that involve assessment, evaluation, or your own nursing judgment. On the exam and in the real world, these duties fall squarely on your shoulders. Make sure that you take primary responsibility for assessing and evaluating the client and for making decisions about the client's care. Never hand off those responsibilities to someone with less training.

Calling in reinforcements

Deciding when to notify a doctor, a social worker, or another hospital staff member is an important element of nursing care. On the exam, however, choices that involve notifying the doctor are usually incorrect. Remember that this exam wants to see you, the nurse, at work.

If you're sure the correct answer is to notify the doctor, make sure that the client's safety has been addressed before notifying a doctor or another staff member. On the exam, the client's safety has a higher priority than notifying other health care providers.

> You can delegate tasks or refer to the doctor, but remember that this exam wants to see the nurse at work!

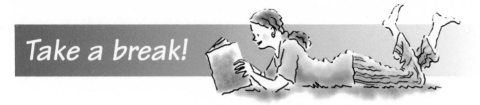

Take a break!

At a crossroads

Completing this crossword puzzle will help you become familiar with concepts related to the NCLEX®. Answers are on the next page.

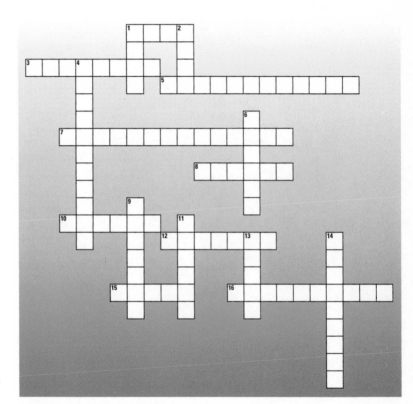

Across

1. The standard multiple-choice question on your licensing exam has this number of possible answers.

3. The exam is a computer-
_____ test.

5. The exam is defined as this type of test.

7. This type of exam question asks you to supply the answer (four words).

8. Each question on the exam is assigned a category based on these needs.

10. _____ , breathing, circulation

12. Using this process may provide insights into helping you analyze a question.

15. The number of times you should read an exam question.

16. Involves coordinating the efforts of other health care workers to provide effective care to your client

Down

1. The number of question formats currently on the exam

2. This is a physiologic need.

4. The most basic needs of all

6. Given high priority on the exam

9. Knowledge of this theory can be a vital tool for establishing priorities on the exam.

11. Writers of the exam

13. The test you must pass to get your nursing license

14. Involved in therapeutic communication

Answer key

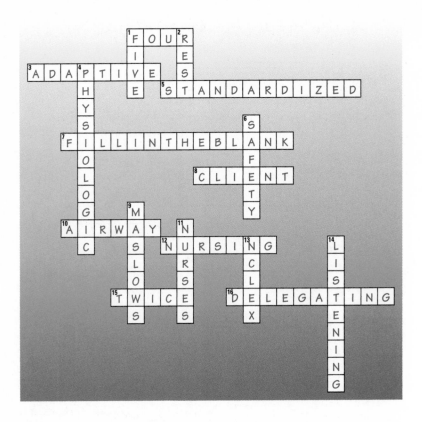

Passing the NCLEX®

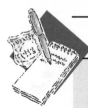

Just the facts

In this chapter, you'll learn:

♦ how to properly prepare for the NCLEX®

♦ how to concentrate during difficult study times

♦ how to make more effective use of your time

♦ how creative studying strategies can enhance learning.

Study preparations

If you're like most people preparing to take the NCLEX®, you're probably feeling nervous, anxious, or concerned. Keep in mind that most test-takers pass the first time around.

Passing the test won't happen by accident, however; you'll need to prepare carefully and efficiently. To help jump-start your preparations:

• determine your strengths and weaknesses
• create a study schedule
• set realistic goals
• find an effective study space
• find creative ways to study
• think positively.

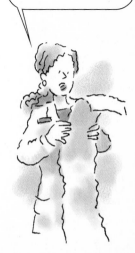

Studying for the exam can seem overwhelming until you break it down into manageable parts.

Strengths and weaknesses

Most students recognize that, even at the end of their nursing studies, they know more about some topics than others. Because the exam covers a broad range of material, you should make some decisions about how intensively you'll review each topic.

Making a list...

Base those decisions on a list. Divide a sheet of paper in half vertically. On one side, list topics you think you know well. On the other side, list topics you feel less secure about. Pay no attention if one side is longer than the other. When you're done studying, you'll feel strong in every area.

...checking it twice

To make sure that your list reflects a comprehensive view of all the areas you studied in school, look at the contents page in the front of this book. For each topic listed, place it in the "know well" column or "needs review" column. Separating content areas this way shows immediately which topics need less study time and which need more.

Scheduling study time

Most people can identify a period of the day when they feel most alert; that's the best time to study. If you feel most alert and energized in the morning, for example, set aside sections of time in the morning for topics that need a lot of review. Then you can use the evening to study topics for which you just need some refreshing. The opposite is true as well; if you're more alert in the evening, study difficult topics at that time.

The great countdown

Set up a basic schedule for studying. Using a calendar or organizer, determine how much time remains before you take the exam. (See *2 to 3 months before the NCLEX®*.) Fill in the remaining days with specific times and topics to be studied. For example, you might schedule the respiratory system on a Tuesday morning and the GI system that afternoon. Remember to schedule difficult topics during your most alert times.

Keep in mind that you shouldn't fill each day with studying. Be realistic and set aside time for normal activities. Try to allow ample study time before the exam and then stick to the schedule.

Realistic goals

Part of creating a schedule means setting goals you can accomplish. You no doubt studied a great deal in nursing school, and by now you have a sense of your own capabilities. Ask yourself, "How much can I cover in a day?" Set that amount of time aside and then stay on task. You'll feel better about yourself — and your chances of passing the exam — when you meet your goals regularly.

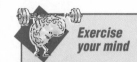
Exercise your mind

2 to 3 months before the NCLEX®

With 2 to 3 months remaining before you plan to take the examination, take these steps:
• Establish a study schedule. Set aside ample time to study, but also leave time for social activities, exercise, family and personal responsibilities, and other matters.
• Become knowledgeable about the exam, its content, the types of questions it asks, and the testing format.
• Begin studying your notes, texts, and other study materials.
• Answer some exam practice questions to help you identify strengths and weaknesses as well as to become familiar with NCLEX®-style questions.

Optimum study time

When you were creating your schedule, you might have asked yourself, "How long should I study? One hour at a stretch? Two hours? Three?" To make the best use of your study time, you'll need to answer those questions.

From beginning to end

Experts are divided about the optimum length of study time. Some say you should study no more than 1 hour at a time several times per day. Their reasoning: You remember the material you study at the beginning and end of a session best, and tend to remember less material studied in the middle of the session.

Other experts say you should hold longer study sessions because you lose time in the beginning, when you're just getting warmed up, and again at the end, when you're cooling down. Therefore, say those experts, a long, concentrated study period will allow you to cover more material.

To thine own self be true

So what's the answer? It doesn't matter as long as you determine what's best for you. At the beginning of your licensing exam study schedule, try study periods of varying lengths. Pay close attention to those that seem more successful.

Remember that you're a trained nurse who is competent at assessment. Think of yourself as a patient, and assess your own progress. Then implement the strategy that works best for you.

Study space

Find a space conducive to effective learning and then study there. Whatever you do, don't study with a television or loud radio on in the room. Instead, find an inviting study space that:
• is located in a quiet, convenient place, away from normal traffic patterns
• contains a solid chair that encourages good posture (Avoid studying in bed; you'll be more likely to fall asleep and not accomplish your goals.)
• has comfortable, soft lighting with which you can see clearly without eye strain
• has a temperature between 65° and 70° F
• contains flowers or green plants, familiar photos or paintings, and easy access to soft, instrumental background music.

Accentuate the positive

Consider taping positive messages around your study space. Make signs with words of encouragement, such as, "You can do it!" "Keep studying!" and "Remember the goal!" These upbeat mes-

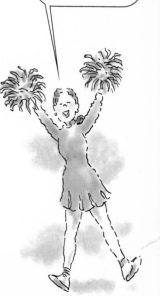

Approach your studying with enthusiasm, sincerity, and determination. It also helps to be awake!

sages can help keep you going when your attention begins to waver.

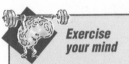

Maintaining concentration

When you're faced with reviewing the amount of information covered by the exam, it's easy to become distracted and lose your concentration. When you lose concentration, you make less effective use of valuable study time. To stay focused, keep these tips in mind:

• Alternate the order of the subjects you study during the day to add variety. Try alternating between topics you find most interesting and those you find least interesting.

• Approach your studying with enthusiasm, sincerity, and determination.

• After you've decided to study, begin immediately. Don't let anything interfere with your thought processes after you've begun.

• Concentrate on accomplishing one task at a time, to the exclusion of everything else.

• Don't try to do two things at once, such as studying and watching television or conversing with friends.

• Work continuously without interruption for a while, but don't study for such a long period that the whole experience becomes grueling or boring.

• Allow time for periodic breaks to give yourself a change of pace. Use these breaks to ease your transition into studying a new topic.

• When studying in the evening, wind down from your studies slowly. Don't progress directly from studying to sleeping.

Taking care of yourself

Never neglect your physical and mental well-being in favor of longer study hours. Maintaining physical and mental health are critical for success in taking the exam. (See *4 to 6 weeks before the exam*.)

A few simple rules

You can increase your likelihood of passing the test by following these simple health rules:

• Get plenty of rest. You can't think deeply or concentrate for long periods when you're tired.

• Eat nutritious meals. Maintaining your energy level is impossible when you're undernourished.

• Exercise regularly. Regular exercise helps you work harder and think more clearly. As a result,

Exercise your mind

4 to 6 weeks before the exam

With 4 to 6 weeks remaining before you plan to take the examination, take these steps:

• Focus on areas of weakness. That way, you'll have time to review these areas again before the test date.

• Find a study partner or form a study group.

• Take a practice test to gauge your skill level early.

• Take time to eat, sleep, exercise, and socialize to avoid burnout.

Kowabonga! Regular exercise helps you work harder and think more clearly.

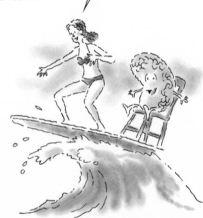

you'll study more efficiently and increase the likelihood of success on the all-important exam.

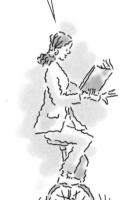

Studying getting dull? Get creative and liven it up.

Memory powers, activate!

If you're having trouble concentrating but would rather push through than take a break, try making your studying more active by reading aloud. Active studying can renew your powers of concentration. By reading review material aloud to yourself, you're engaging your ears as well as your eyes — and making your studying a more active process. Hearing the material aloud also fosters memory and subsequent recall.

You can also rewrite in your own words a few of the more difficult concepts you're reviewing. Explaining these concepts in writing forces you to think through the material and can jump-start your memory.

Creative studying

Even when you study in a perfect study space and concentrate better than ever, studying for the exam can get a little, well, dull. Even people with terrific study habits occasionally feel bored or sluggish. That's why it's important to have some creative tricks in your study bag to liven up your studying during these down times.

Creative studying doesn't have to be hard work. It involves making efforts to alter your study habits a bit. Some techniques that might help include making use of short study sessions, studying with a partner or group, and creating flash cards or other audiovisual study tools.

Quick study

We all have spaces in our day that might otherwise be dead time. (See *1 week before the exam.*) These are perfect times to review for the exam but not to cover new material because, by the time you get deep into new material, your time will be over. Always keep some flash cards or a small notebook handy for situations when you have a few extra minutes.

You'll be amazed how many short sessions you can find in a day and how much reviewing you can do in 5 minutes. These occasions offer short stretches of time you can use for studying:
• eating breakfast
• waiting for or riding on a train or bus
• waiting in line at the bank, post office, bookstore, or other places.

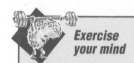

Exercise your mind

1 week before the exam

With 1 week remaining before the examination, take these steps:
• Take a review test to measure your progress.
• Record key ideas and principles on note cards or audiotapes.
• Rest, eat well, and avoid thinking about the examination during non-study times.
• Treat yourself to one special event. You've been working hard, and you deserve it!

Study partners

Studying with a partner or group of students can be an excellent way to energize your studying. Working with a partner allows you to test each other on the material you've reviewed. Your partner can give you encouragement and motivation. Perhaps most important, working with a partner can provide a welcome break from solitary studying.

The perfect partner

Exercise some care when choosing a study partner or assembling a study group. A partner who doesn't fit your needs won't help you make the most of your study time. Look for a partner who:

• possesses goals similar to yours. For example, someone taking the exam at approximately the same date who feels the same sense of urgency as you do might make an excellent partner.

• possesses roughly the same level of knowledge as you. Tutoring someone can sometimes help you learn, but partnering should be give-and-take so both partners can gain knowledge.

• can study without excess chatting or interruptions. Socializing is an important part of creative study but, remember, you still have to pass the exam — so stay serious!

Audiovisual tools

Using CD-ROMs, flash cards, and other audiovisual tools fosters retention and makes learning and reviewing fun.

CD-ROM — it's the bomb!

CD-ROMs provide an audiovisual format that allows the learner to apply her knowledge and receive immediate feedback. CD-ROMs present nursing information and case studies and simulate clinical situations through an interactive medium. These products are available on many nursing topics. You'll even find CD-ROMs that specifically address exam preparation and include sample test questions.

Better late than never

If you weren't required to use CD-ROMs during your nursing education, this is a great time to start. Check out the CD-ROM included with this book. You can also check the library of your nursing school for CD-ROMs to borrow or use on the premises, or purchase your own online or at your local bookstore or school's bookstore.

Flash Gordon? No, it's Flash Card!

Flash cards can provide you with an excellent study tool. The process of writing material on a flash card will help you remember it. In addition, flash cards are small and portable, making them perfect for those 5-minute slivers of time that show up during the day.

Creating a flash card should be fun. Use magic markers, high-lighters, and other colorful tools to make them visually stimulating. The more effort you put into creating your flash cards, the better you'll remember the material written on the cards.

Picture this!

Flowcharts, drawings, diagrams, and other image-oriented study aids can also help you learn material more effectively. Substituting images for text can be a great way to give your eyes a break and recharge your brain. Remember to use vivid colors to make your creations visually engaging.

The ears have it

If you learn more effectively when you hear information rather than see it, consider recording key ideas using a handheld tape recorder. Recording information helps promote memory because you say the information aloud when taping and then listen to it when playing it back. Like flash cards, tapes are portable and perfect for those short study periods during the day. (See *The day before the exam*.)

Check your attitude

Positive thinking is more than a cliché for a greeting card; it's a bonafide technique for enhancing your chances of success.

Saying is believing

As the clock ticks down to that all-important moment, think about all the hard work you've done and all the material you've learned. Tell yourself that you're ready and that you can do it. You might even want to plan a post-examination celebration. Giving yourself some well-deserved words of encouragement will help you walk into the testing room with a positive, confident attitude.

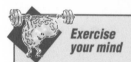

Exercise your mind

The day before the exam

With 1 day before the examination, take these steps:

• Drive to the test site, review traffic patterns, and find out where to park. If your route to the test site takes you through heavy traffic or if you're expecting bad weather, set aside extra time to ensure prompt arrival.

• Do something relaxing during the day.

• Rest, eat well, and avoid dwelling on the exam during nonstudy periods.

• Call a supportive friend or relative for some last-minute words of encouragement.

• Avoid your classmates who may be nervous or excessively jittery about the exam because they'll only increase your anxiety.

Practice questions

Practice questions should be an important part of your study strategy. Practice questions can improve your studying by helping you review material and familiarizing yourself with the exact style of questions you'll encounter on the exam.

Never put off 'til tomorrow

Consider working through some practice questions as soon as you begin studying for the exam. For example, you might try a few of the questions that appear at the end of each chapter in this book.

If you do well, you probably know the material contained in that chapter fairly well and can spend less time reviewing that particular topic. If you have trouble with the questions, spend extra study time on that topic.

I'm getting there

Practice questions also can provide an excellent means of marking your progress. Don't worry if you have trouble answering the first few practice questions you try; you'll need time to adjust to the way the questions are asked. Eventually you'll become accustomed to the question format and you'll begin to focus more on the questions themselves.

If you make practice questions a regular part of your study regimen, you'll be able to notice areas in which you're improving. You can then adjust your study time accordingly.

Practice makes perfect

As you near the examination date, you should increase the number of practice questions you answer at one sitting. This will enable you to approximate the experience of taking the actual examination. Using the CD-ROM found at the back of this book, you can take practice tests of 10, 25, 50, or 75 questions. Note that 75 questions is the minimum number of questions you'll be asked on the actual examination. By gradually tackling larger practice tests, you'll increase your confidence, build test-taking endurance, and strengthen the concentration skills that enable you to succeed on the exam. (See *The day of the exam.*)

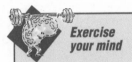

Exercise your mind

The day of the exam

On the day of the examination, take these steps:
• Get up early.
• Wear comfortable clothes, preferably with layers, so you can adjust to fit the room temperature.
• Leave your house early.
• Arrive at the test site early.
• Avoid looking at your notes as you wait for your test computer.
• Listen carefully to the instructions given before entering the test room.
• Stay confident and positive, and have faith in yourself.
  Good luck!

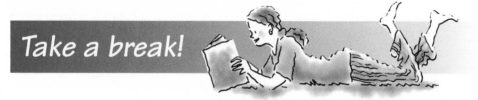

Take a break!

Another kind of quiz...

Need a break from studying? Try your hand at these "sample" questions! Hint: Have fun! Answers are on the next page.

1. When is the best time to study?
    A. While you're watching your favorite soap opera
    B. When you're alert and free from distraction
    C. When you're talking to your mom on the phone
    D. Late at night, when you're exhausted

2. Which description illustrates the perfect study space?
    A. Sitting on the cold cement floor in the hallway of your dorm
    B. Lying in your bed at night, under the covers, using a flashlight to see
    C. Sitting at a tidy desk in a quiet room with natural lighting
    D. In your car (while driving) on the way to the exam

3. What isn't considered an effective audiovisual tool for studying?
    A. Using colorful flash cards
    B. Using interactive CD-ROMs
    C. Creating easy-to-understand flowcharts
    D. Writing on the palm of your hand

4. What should you do the night before the exam?
    A. Call your best friend to catch up.
    B. Study for the exam all night — don't even sleep!
    C. Continually tell yourself that there's no way you'll pass.
    D. Unplug your alarm clock to see if you'll be able to wake up for the test on your own!

5. What should you do the morning of the test?
    A. Squeeze yourself into the tightest pair of jeans you can find, and head off to the test.
    B. A half-hour before the test begins, look on a map and try to figure out just where this test center is located!
    C. Pack all your study aids so you can study right up until the test begins.
    D. Eat a good breakfast, arrive at the test site early, take a deep breath, and tell yourself that you can do it!

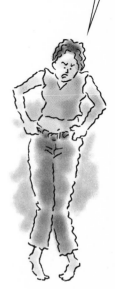

Maybe this wasn't such a good idea...

Answer key

1. The answer is B.
If you must see today's episode of *Days of our Lives,* watch it during a study break! Call Mom after your studying is finished (she'd want it that way!), and remember to study when you're well-rested.

2. The answer is C.
Try not to study in high-traffic areas, like your dorm hallway — and the open road! Lying in bed while studying at night will only cause you to wake up with crinkled papers under your face and highlighter in your hair!

3. The answer is D.
Save your palms for clapping for yourself and toasting your victory after you pass the exam!

4. The answer is A.
Relax! Be prepared for the test, but don't stress over it. Make sure that you spend time resting. A chat with a friend can give you the support you need and take your mind off the exam.

5. The answer is D.
Be smart! Dress well, plan ahead, and avoid cramming right before the examination. You've studied hard — be confident!

11

Success as a new graduate

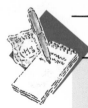

Just the facts

In this chapter, you'll learn:

♦ how to create a resumé

♦ interview techniques

♦ ways to work with your preceptor

♦ tips for a smooth orientation to your new job.

Searching for a job

Well, you finally made it. As you walk down the aisle past your fellow graduates, you see the smiling faces of your friends and family, and reality finally hits you. Soon, the next phase of your career will begin, and it can be as challenging (and rewarding) as school has been. The first step of this new phase is searching for a job.

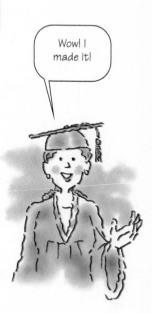

Wow! I made it!

Who, what, where, when, why?

Make sure you know what you want before you start looking for a position. Where do you want to practice? Do you want to practice in an acute setting such as a hospital? Are you interested in long-term care, home care, or a clinic or community setting? Do you know where you want your career to be in 5 years? Are you going to continue your education? After you narrow your focus, your search can begin.

Creating a resumé

The first step in the application process is your formal introduction to the hospital (or other health care setting) via your resumé. A clear, concise cover letter and a well-organized, professional resumé are essential; together, they're the first step toward acquiring a position.

Wonderful me!

Remember this: writing your resumé shouldn't be an exercise in modesty. It may be hard to get used to the idea, but this is the time to toot your own horn and show prospective employers why they should hire *you* rather than someone else!

Cover letter

The cover letter is the first piece of information an employer sees. A well-written cover letter will make the employer want to find out more about you and lead them to read your resumé. Conversely, a cover letter that appears unprofessional or unclear may make the employer wonder why she should spend more of her valuable time reading your resumé.

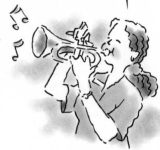

Tooting your own horn is definitely permitted during your job search. So, toot away on your resumé!

The letter must be concise and should quickly capture the recruiter's attention. If your cover letter is too long, the recruiter won't get to the resumé! Two to three single-spaced paragraphs is the standard length.

Dear specific person...

Begin your letter by addressing a specific person, making sure the spelling of the name, title, and credentials is correct. If you can't get the spelling from an advertisement, call the recruitment office to verify this information.

I need a job...

Next, state the purpose of your letter, referring to the title of the position you're seeking and how you heard about it. The next paragraph should present your qualifications as they relate to the position you're seeking.

...and there's more!

Lastly, close the letter with an offer to provide additional information if necessary, and your desire to hear from the recruiter. One final tip—always mail or fax a cover letter with the resumé. A cover letter or resumé sent alone isn't helpful for the recruiter and will most likely receive no response. (See *Sample cover letter.*)

Parts of a resumé

A resumé is a summary of your education, experience, and qualifications. It's your introduction to a prospective employer. You only get one chance to make a first impression, so your resumé must be organized, clearly written, and an example of the professionalism you'll show on the job. (See *Resumé do's and don'ts.*)

Sample cover letter

Here's an example of a clear, concise, well-written cover letter. Remember that the cover letter forms a prospective employer's first impression of you and may determine whether she thinks it's worth her time to look at your resumé!

June 30, 2005

Jane Carter
1234 American Street
Smithville, MA 12221
(123) 456-7890 (Home)
(123) 098-7654 (Cellular)

Mary Jones, RN, MSN
Nurse Recruiter
Jamesville Hospital
789 11th Street
Jamesville, MA 12343

Ms. Jones,

I am responding to your advertisement for Medical Surgical Nurses that appeared in the February issue of *Nursing 2005*. I believe that my education and work experience have prepared me for this position. I have enclosed a copy of my resumé for your review.

I look forward to learning more about Jamesville Hospital and the possibility of becoming a member of your team. Thank you for your consideration.

Sincerely,

Jane Carter

Jane Carter

Enclosure: Resume

Advice from the experts

Resumé do's and don'ts

Use these tips to write an effective resumé.

Do's
- Be clear.
- Be concise.
- Be honest.
- Include honors and awards and volunteer work.
- Include a cover letter.
- Use high-quality bond paper (white or cream).
- Stay consistent and organized in overall appearance and content.
- Use the Times New Roman font in 12 point type.
- Review your resumé and cover letter carefully for grammar and spelling errors.

Don'ts
- Don't rely on spell check; instead, read over your resumé and cover letter carefully (and ask a friend to read it, too).
- Don't use fancy or unreadable fonts.
- Don't use colored paper or colored print.
- Don't handwrite on the resumé.

Less is more

For new graduates, a one-page resumé is sufficient. If your resumé becomes longer than two pages, review it carefully and try to edit out unnecessary information. It's important to remember that the recruiter should be able to scan your resumé quickly.

There are many different types and styles of resumés, but each resumé should include these essential components, in this order:
- demographic information
- education
- work experience (nursing, related and unrelated)
- professional achievements (including honors and awards)
- professional and academic memberships
- related personal and volunteer activities. (See *Sample resumé*.)

Demographics

The demographic section should include your name, address, telephone number, cellular phone number, and e-mail address. If you don't have a professional-sounding e-mail address you may want to change it, at least temporarily. You might also want to change the message on your answering machine or cell phone.

Education

After the demographic section is a summary of your education. Begin with your most recent degree or diploma, and be sure to include honors or awards you've received. Be sure to include the school name, city, and state for each school you attended. If you haven't graduated yet, include the expected date of graduation.

Work experience

The next section of the resumé describes your work experience. Again, list your employment in reverse chronological order, beginning with your current or most recent position. Be sure to include the facility or employer name, city and state, job title, and dates of employment. Under each position you may include a few bullets that identify accomplishments and leadership responsibilities of that position.

A stroll down memory lane

Don't forget to include positions held outside nursing and health if you feel they point to strengths that would be assets to your nursing career. Think back to your college years and even to high school. Did you spend a summer working as a camp counselor for children with special needs? Did you have an after-school job as a pharmacy assistant?

> Think back to your school days when you write your resumé. An interesting after-school job may be just the thing to catch a prospective employer's eye!

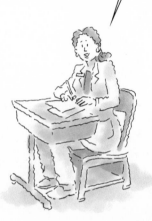

Sample resumé

Jane Carter

1234 American Street
Smithville, MA 12221
(123) 456-7890

janecarter@email.com

EDUCATION
09/00 – 06/04   Bachelor of Science in Nursing
Hilltop University, Johnston, Massachusetts

EXPERIENCE
05/02 – Present Nursing Extern
Massachusetts General Hospital
Boston, Massachusetts

09/00 – 04/02   Certified Nursing Assistant
Jones Nursing Home
Smithville, Massachusetts

HONORS/AWARDS
Dean's List, 2002, Hilltop University
National Student Nurses Association Scholarship
awarded 2003

MEMBERSHIPS
Sigma Theta Tau International
National Student Nurses' Association

CERTIFICATIONS
Basic Cardiac Life Support (BCLS)

COMMUNITY ACTIVITIES
Volunteer at the local Red Cross Blood Drive

Professional achievements

In the professional achievement section, bragging is allowed! As in previous sections of the resumé, the items in this section should be listed in reverse chronological order, from most to least recent.

Mom would be so proud!

Did you receive special honors in nursing school? Perhaps you were awarded an "employee of the month" award at a previous job. Maybe you even helped to write or research a paper that was published or were selected as a professor's research assistant.

Professional and academic memberships

Listing professional and academic memberships shows prospective employers that you're truly interested in learning about and becoming involved in your chosen field.

No shortcuts!

Completely spell out the full name of any association and avoid the use of abbreviations, such as ANA or SNA. List licensures or certifications under a separate heading.

Community and volunteer services

Lastly, include a section on personal activities, such as community or volunteer services. Providing this information will show the potential employer that you're a well-rounded individual. It will also provide some insight into your personality and augment your resumé if you lack work experience.

A helping hand

Volunteer work may be a person's first exposure to the "working world." We learn a lot from volunteering, and prospective employers learn that you're a caring, compassionate person who wants to make a difference (one definition of a good nurse).

Optional information

Depending on your experience, you may want to include some additional information on your resumé, including references, clinical experience, and honors and awards that aren't directly related to your nursing career.

References

Most employers will assume that you'll provide references but, even if it isn't required, you may choose to include a line on your resumé that states, "References available upon request." If the guidelines for application request that you include professional references, you may provide them on a separate sheet.

Most employers who request references ask that you provide three. Be sure to contact your references first; never list someone as a reference without getting their permission.

Clinical experience

Some new graduates include their nursing school clinical experience in their resumés; however, if the clinical experience section makes your resumé longer than two pages, leave it out.

Honors and awards

Record honors, awards, grants, scholarships, and programs that allowed you to study abroad in a separate section. Be sure to list only those awards that you haven't already listed in the professional achievements section. In addition, include academic awards you received while attending school only if you're a new graduate; most employers aren't interested in "ancient history."

Some things are better left unsaid

Some items that should be omitted from your resumé are references to marital status, age, race, or religion. Although the potential employer may be interested to know your hobbies, they shouldn't be listed on your resumé. Remember, the reader should be able to scan your resumé and find the relevant information in no more than 30 seconds.

> Employers should be blind to your marital status, number of children, age, race, and religion. Be sure to leave those details out of your resumé.

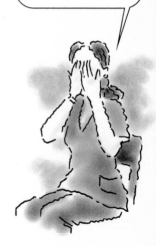

Interview techniques

Your beautifully written, professional cover letter and resumé got you "in the door" and you've been called to schedule an interview! Check your calendar carefully and be flexible when scheduling the date for the interview. This scheduling call will be your would-be employer's first impression of your flexibility as a potential staff member. Try to select a date and time when you won't be rushed or exhausted.

No excuses!

You should arrive at your interview on time (or a bit early), looking professional, well rested, and enthusiastic. Your prospective employer isn't interested in excuses; she wants to know that you're taking this opportunity seriously.

What to wear, what to wear?

After you've scheduled your interview, take a look at your wardrobe. You don't need an expensive business suit to make a good impression; just make sure your clothes are clean and pressed, keep jewelry to a minimum and tasteful, and don't wear overpowering cologne or perfume. If you have a tattoo, you may want to wear clothing that covers it. Remove nose rings, eyebrow rings, or other jewelry that may be distracting. Just think "professional appearance" and you can't go wrong. (See *Interviewing do's and don'ts.*)

Preparing for questions

The point of the interview (from the employer's perspective) is to learn as much about the potential candidate as possible, so get ready to answer questions. To prepare for the interview, take some time to research the facility; most have a Web site. Take a look at the site and become familiar with the facility's mission. Carry a small portfolio or binder with an additional copy of your resumé and references. All these tips will help you appear prepared and professional!

To prepare for questions from the recruiters, remember that the questions are usually open-ended and probing to test your problem-solving and clinical-thinking skills. These questions will also focus on your introspective view of nursing as a profession. Your answers should be brief, articulate, and honest.

Mirror, mirror, on the wall

To prepare, try sitting in front of a mirror and practicing some responses to such questions as:
• Why did you decide to become a nurse?
• What type of nursing are you interested in? Why?
• What did you enjoy most about nursing school? Least?
• How did your experiences in school help prepare you for your nursing career?
• What is it about you that will make you a good nurse?
• What are your strengths? What areas need improvement?

Do you measure up?

You might even tape your answers and then try to listen to them with an objective ear. It's also helpful to ask someone who has already been through a successful interview to role-play the employer and critique you on your responses.

Do your responses really answer the questions being asked? Do you answer the question right away or does it take a while for you to get to the point? Are your answers concise and articulate or wordy and unclear? If you aren't happy with your responses, simply practice some more.

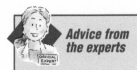

Advice from the experts

Interviewing do's and don'ts

These tips will help you make the best possible first impression during your all-important job interview.

Do's
• Be prepared by creating a list of questions you want to ask and developing answers to questions the recruiter might ask.
• Take a test run to the facility.
• Dress professionally.
• Arrive early and check your appearance in a mirror.
• Bring the name and phone number of the person you're meeting.
• Bring a few extra copies of your resumé.
• Bring a list of references and their contact information.

Don'ts
• Don't wear excessive jewelry or makeup.
• Don't chew gum.
• Don't complain about the parking.
• Don't complain about your former employer.

Supercalifragilistic...not!

Interviewers aren't impressed by large words; they're impressed by candidates who can think on their feet and reply clearly and honestly in a professional, yet relaxed demeanor (all qualities of a good nurse, by the way). Be sure to maintain eye contact during the interview; look directly at the recruiter while answering questions.

Off-limits

Remember that there are questions that shouldn't be asked by a potential employer—questions you don't have to answer. In fact, in the era of equal opportunity employment, it's illegal for potential employers to discuss certain topics. These include questions regarding your race, marital status, future plans to have children, age, religion, and national origin. If you're asked these questions and you don't feel comfortable answering them, you could say, "I was told I wouldn't need to discuss those issues, but I'm glad to talk with you about anything related to nursing."

While you prepare to answer the interviewer's questions, prepare some questions of your own. You can keep a copy of the questions in your portfolio and jot down the answers as you receive them. (See *Questions to consider asking*.)

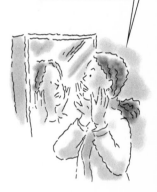

Writing a follow-up letter or two can keep our name and face fresh in the minds of potential employers. Well there's a fresh face!

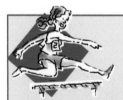

Overcoming obstacles

Questions to consider asking

Nervous about interviewing for a job? See if this student's question sounds familiar.

Question

I always draw a blank when an interviewer asks if I have questions. What should I ask?

Words of wisdom

Here are some questions you might want to ask during an interview:

• Are there opportunities for continuing education activities, including additional certifications?

• What does the orientation program consist of, and does it include a mentoring program?

• Upon completion of my orientation, how many patients will I care for on a shift?

• Is there shift differential?

• Will I be required to float to other units if they're short-staffed?

• Does the hospital have a mandatory overtime policy?

• Will I have rotating shifts between days and nights, days and evenings, etc?

• What's the leadership style on the unit?

• What level of patient acuity can I expect?

• What are the current goals for the unit?

• What are the staffing needs on this unit?

• What's the greatest need on this unit?

• I'm going to continue my nursing education. Is there flexibility within my work schedule?

Ah, relief!

As you breathe a sigh of relief and drive home from the interview, remember, there's one more task to complete. As soon as you arrive home, write a follow-up letter to the recruiter, thanking her for the opportunity to interview and your interest in the position. If you had the opportunity to meet the nurse-manager, consider sending a note to her as well.

Transitioning to your new role

It has finally happened. All your hard work has paid off and you've been hired for the position. Congratulations! Now you must prepare for an entirely new experience.

Transitioning to a new role as a nurse can be a challenging — and exciting — experience. You've been a student for a while, but this time of transition should also be considered a learning experience. You may feel overwhelmed with the amount of information you receive during your first weeks in your new position, but everything will eventually click.

Give yourself a break!

The number-one rule is to be patient with yourself. Give yourself time to absorb the information. The first few days will be general facility orientation and may include the computer system, fire safety, infection control, general policies and procedures, and human resource information. Because the orientation may include other newly hired employees, the scope of this component of the orientation may be broad. If you need to be recertified in basic cardiac life support (BCLS), this may also take place during your orientation period.

Sharpen your pencil!

After the general facility orientation, a general nursing orientation will take place. Nursing policy and procedures will be reviewed. Drug calculation and medication administration tests may be given. Take notes during the orientation; you may have some homework to do! You may need to refresh your memory with some procedures and learn new policies and procedures specific to the facility.

Although each unit follows the general facility policy and procedures manuals, specific units may have individualized manuals. Take some time to review the policies and procedures manual for your specific unit because it contains specific guidelines on all the procedures you'll be expected to perform.

The homestretch!

Now you're ready and finally arrive on your unit. Come prepared; bring your stethoscope, name tag, scissors, penlight, pens, and a drug reference. If you have a small calculator, that will be useful as well. You may also wish to consider a pocket personal data organizer with references if you have the financial resources. Last but not least, be prepared to meet a lot of new people.

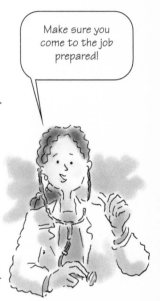

Make sure you come to the job prepared!

Meeting your nurse-manager

The nurse-manager is the person in charge. You may have had the opportunity to meet her during your interview, or you may have been hired by the nurse-manager. Remember that the nurse-manager has 24-hour accountability for the unit and is responsible for staffing, patient care, budgeting, patient and family complaints, staffing issues, conflict resolution, and overall management of the unit.

Getting to know you...

After you begin your new job, the manager may request an individual meeting with you to reintroduce herself and to check on your progress. This is her opportunity to get to know you on a one-on-one basis.

...getting to know all about you

She may want to hear your goals, your progress in orientation, and plans for your career. She may review what's expected of you and where she sees you fitting in on the unit. You can ask about your evaluation process and if your nurse-manager has other standards that she looks at in addition to the facility's evaluation.

It's important to discuss with the nurse-manager the best way to meet with her. Does she prefer that you schedule an appointment or does she have an "open-door policy" that invites you to stop by her office informally? It's also important to identify the management style of the nurse-manager, which will make working with her much easier. (See *Leadership role of the nurse-manager*, page 218.)

I'm all ears!

Remember, this meeting is an opportunity for the nurse-manager to assess you as a team member. Try to concentrate on listening to what she has to say.

> ## Leadership role of the nurse-manager
>
> The nurse-manager assumes 24-hour accountability for the nursing care delivered in a specific nursing area. Different nurse-managers have different leadership styles. Knowing your nurse-manager's professional style will help you to work with her more effectively.
>
> **Management styles**
> - *Autocratic*—The manager makes decisions with little or no staff input and doesn't delegate responsibility. Staff dependence is fostered.
> - *Laissez-faire*—The manager provides little direction, structure, or support and abdicates responsibility and decision making when possible. Staff development isn't facilitated. There's little interest in achieving the goals necessary for adequate patient care.
> - *Democratic*—The manager encourages staff members to participate in decision making when possible. Most decisions are made by the group. Staff development is encouraged. The manager carefully delegates responsibilities and gives feedback to staff members to encourage professional growth.
> - *Participative*—The manager identifies problems and presents them to the staff with possible solutions. Staff members are encouraged to provide input, but the manager makes the decision. Negotiation is key. The manager encourages staff advancement.

Standards of care

Standards of care are the guidelines that nurses use daily in all aspects of care; they form the basis for competent care. They're established as a way to provide safe, effective care. Standards vary according to the type of care and who's providing the care. In addition, the facility or agency is periodically evaluated by an accrediting body that assesses the services and providers to determine it's in compliance with established standards of care.

When in doubt, look it up!

In every facility, there's a procedure manual on each unit. This manual contains the standards of care for every component of nursing care. It outlines policies and procedures and should be reviewed during your orientation. A *policy* is an overall plan to accomplish goals, and a *procedure* is the tool used to implement the policy. Never hesitate to "look it up" if you're unsure.

Fitting in on the unit

You're the new kid on the block. Take a few days to get used to the layout of the unit, the locker room, the staff assignment board, and the medication room. It's also important to determine the type of system the unit follows to deliver patient care. Understanding the type of delivery system will help you better understand your role and responsibilities as a nurse as well as the responsibilities of the other staff members. (See *Understanding delivery systems.*)

The best advice to the new person is to observe, observe, observe—and be prepared. Arrive 10 minutes early so you have time to gather your equipment and mentally prepare for the day.

Personality type — "be positive"

Be friendly and have a positive attitude. Try to be the first person to say hello to the others in the morning. Focus on leaving personal business at home and limit personal phone calls to break time.

Don't be a complainer. You'll encounter negative people in the workplace who will give you an earful on

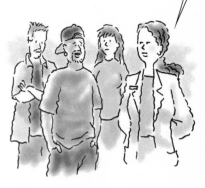

You may feel 15 again. Fitting in can be a challenge when you're the "new kid on the block." Just give it time; soon you'll be the person that other "new kids" come to for advice!

Understanding delivery systems

The members of each nursing unit choose a delivery system that best meets the needs of their patients. The delivery systems listed here are most commonly used today:

• *Team nursing*—A registered nurse (RN) leads nursing staff who work together to provide care for a specific number of patients. The team typically consists of RNs, licensed practical nurses (LPNs), and patient-care attendants. The team leader assesses patient needs, plans patient care, and revises the care plan based on changes in the patient's condition. The team leader assigns tasks to team members as needed.

• *Modular nursing*—Modular nursing is similar to team nursing, but the team is typically smaller. An RN is assigned to a group of patients in a specific geographic location. Typically, an RN is paired with an LPN to care for a small group of patients.

• *Primary nursing*—An RN plans and organizes care for a group of patients and cares for this group during their entire hospitalization. The RN assumes 24-hour accountability for this group of patients. She delegates care in her absence to other staff members. An RN who cares for the patients in the absence of the primary nurse is called an *associate nurse*. The associate nurse follows the care plan developed by the primary nurse.

• *Total patient care nursing*—An RN plans, organizes, and delivers patient care for a specific group of patients. If an LPN is caring for a group of patients, an RN assesses the patients and plans the care delivered by the LPN.

• *Functional nursing*—Each caregiver in a specific nursing unit is given specific tasks that fall into her scope of practice. For example, an RN may administer medications to the entire unit, whereas an LPN performs treatments, and the patient-care attendants provide physical care.

• *Case management*—This form of primary nursing involves an RN who manages the care of an assigned group of patients. This nurse coordinates care with the entire health care team. She helps develop protocols, policies, and procedures, and develops a plan to achieve patient outcomes.

the problems related to the unit, facility, or management. You'll also encounter people who are anxious to share the latest gossip about your colleagues. Avoid getting involved, keep an open mind, and maintain a positive attitude.

Ask and you shall receive

Ask questions of your coworkers. Asking questions is a good way to open the lines of communication with your colleagues and show your eagerness to learn. Remember, all nurses were new graduates at one point in their careers.

Off-color is off-limits!

Although it may seem obvious, don't use humor that could be considered racist, sexist, or off-color. Try not to engage in such conversations; simply walk away if the situation occurs.

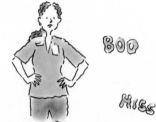

Tough group! I guess this material wouldn't go over too well at work tomorrow.

BOO

BOO

HISS

Working with a preceptor

As a new graduate, you'll be assigned a preceptor who will work with you during your orientation period. The preceptor is usually a staff nurse who has either volunteered to precept or has been asked by management to fulfill this role. This person will guide you through the unit's routine.

Personal and professional goals

You'll have goals established for your orientation; read them carefully. Make a note of goals you think will be more difficult for you, and develop personal goals and share them with your preceptor. If you're aware of your strengths and weaknesses and you share them with your preceptor, she may be able to find additional experiences to help you meet your goals.

You never know unless you ask

Don't be afraid to ask questions or ask for help. It's true that no question is stupid or trivial, and not asking may lead to an error. You won't be expected to jump right into your position and know all the answers. You'll have more questions than answers in the beginning.

Constructive criticism

An essential component of the learning experience is feedback. Typically, regular meetings are scheduled with your preceptor and the nurse-manager to monitor your progress and allow you to discuss your concerns. If progress meetings aren't included in your orientation, ask for them. This shows that you care about your job and your performance.

Thicken up that skin!

Recognize the need to assess your ability to accept constructive criticism during this period. Remember, it's your preceptor's job to orient you to this facility. There will be times that you'll do something wrong and she'll remind you. Try not to take it personally.

As you near the end of your orientation program, you may be asked to evaluate your preceptor and the orientation program. Be honest in your appraisal.

Organizational skills

As you transition from a student nurse to a graduate nurse you may begin to wonder, "was I ever organized?" As a student, you had different responsibilities and, perhaps, a lighter patient load. In addition to prioritizing the needs of multiple patients, you're now expected to monitor your patients' progress, communicate with the other members of the health care team, provide emotional support to patients and families, delegate and supervise ancillary staff, and document, document, document. You're well prepared to fulfill each of these responsibilities, but remember that organization takes time. Be patient and begin using simple solutions.

Taking report

When you take report, use a system that helps you organize the information you receive. Use a multicolored pen to highlight important information, such as laboratory data you're waiting for or the time your patient is scheduled to leave the unit for a diagnostic procedure.

Pen in hand

Allow space on your report sheet to jot down throughout the day any information you'll need to provide a thorough report at the end of your shift. It's impossible to remember everything, and if you begin the habit of writing it down, it will become second nature and your report will be complete every time.

Expect the unexpected!

After report, take a moment to assess your assignment and make a brief action plan. Of course, it's to be expected that unexpected things will occur that change your plan; as a matter of fact, it's inevitable! Just take the time to reassess and formulate another plan for the remainder of the day.

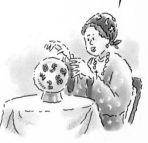

Don't rely on your "supernatural" powers of memory. Pen and paper are much more reliable!

You may find that you're spending more time on a task than is reasonable. Are you delegating all you can? Can you use the secretary on the unit to make phone calls for you? If you have ancillary staff assigned to you, delegate appropriate tasks to them. Also, don't forget to note on your report sheet what information you'll need from your ancillary staff at the end of the day to give a thorough report.

All in a day's work

Give yourself time to develop a routine. Observe experienced nurses on the floor to pick up timesaving and organizational tips. A strong orientation program will include information on prioritizing and organizing your nursing care.

Clinical judgment and decision making

A nurse needs to exercise clinical judgment. To develop sound clinical judgment, you need to use the critical thinking skills you learned in nursing school. Critical thinking is a mixture of knowledge, intuition, logic, common sense, and experience; it improves with increasing clinical skill and scientific experience. (See *Critical thinking: An essential skill.*)

Clinical judgment and on-the-spot decision making are crucial components of nursing. Many factors are involved in making a clinical decision, including knowledge, experience, and situational stressors. The nursing process can serve as a guide as you begin

Critical thinking: An essential skill

In the complex, rapidly changing health care environment, critical thinking is a necessary skill for providing safe, effective nursing care. Critical thinking takes basic problem solving one step further by considering all related factors, including the patient's unique needs as well as any of the nurse's thoughts and beliefs that may influence her decision-making ability. Critical-thinking skills enable the nurse to take a step outside the situation and look at the whole picture more objectively.

Truth seekers
Critical thinkers have the desire to seek truth and actively pursue answers to questions to

obtain this complete picture. They're also open-minded and creative and can draw from past clinical experience to come up with all possible alternatives and then zero in on the best solution for the patient.

Practice for your practice
Books, articles, and online courses are available to hone nurses' critical-thinking skills. When nurses engage in critical thinking, their patients have the best chances for success!

your practice. Following the steps of the nursing process (assessment, diagnosis, planning, implementation, and evaluation) will help you guide your practice and make patient care decisions.

New situations

As you encounter each new situation, assess the data available to you and identify potential concerns. If something doesn't look right, investigate further; you may need to collect and assess more data. When you have the data in hand, set goals, establish your nursing diagnoses, and set priorities. Now is the time to get to work. This is when you undertake the task, or perhaps delegate the task to someone else.

Evaluating care

Lastly, evaluate the care you've provided — directly and by delegation. This process allows you to evaluate the patient's response and modify the care plan to achieve the goals. It's an ongoing process that can be applied to simple or complex problems.

A little help, please

Don't be afraid to ask for help as you assess, diagnose, plan, implement, or evaluate the care you're providing. Use of the nursing process should be the organizing framework from which you work.

Learning from others

Another way to help develop your critical-thinking and clinical-judgment skills is by observing the more seasoned nurses on your unit. Watch their response to emergencies, the ancillary staff, and their patients and families. Although an expert nurse may not be able to explain all the thoughts that went into her particular actions, talking about it may provide you with some guidance. Most experienced nurses are willing to share their expertise and will appreciate the fact that you view them as an expert.

Always, at the end of each day, review your activities. What did you do well, and what could you have done better?

Dealing with emergencies

It's going to happen sooner or later: your first code situation. Don't panic; you aren't alone. You're a member of a team. The code team is a group of experienced professionals who will respond to this emergency.

Know your role

You'll probably review a code situation in your nursing orientation. Many facilities provide a mock code to familiarize you with the facility's procedures for an emergency. Take advantage of this opportunity to listen and learn. Ask questions. Take notes. Know your responsibility in an emergency situation. How do you call a code? Who's on the code team? What's your responsibility during the situation?

Know your patients

It's important for you to know the code status of each of your patients. If it isn't provided during report, take a moment to look at the patient's chart. Make sure that it's documented, and review the facility's policy on advance directives. It's also essential to know where the code cart is located on your unit. It should always stay in the same location unless it's being used for an emergency on your unit.

Know your responsibilities

If you're in a patient's room and he appears to be in distress, don't panic; remember your ABCs (airway, breathing, and circulation). Check to see if the patient is unresponsive. If he isn't responding, open his airway, check for a pulse, and call for help. Begin compressions as you wait for the defibrillator, other emergency equipment, and the code team. Employ the assistance of other nurses and staff to take care of your other patients while you stay with the patient who's experiencing an emergency. During an emergency situation, the team is usually at its best and will pitch in to assist.

> Know where the code cart is located on your unit and make sure it's always in the same location when not in use.

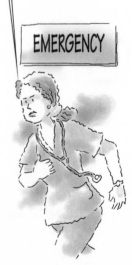

The cavalry arrives!

When the code team arrives, they'll take over. If you have begun compressions, they may offer to take over. Your responsibility will be to relay patient information to the code team. The code will continue until the patient is stabilized or until the team can't revive the patient. The doctor will determine when a patient can't be revived and order code procedures to stop.

Emergency follow-up

Following the code, you'll need to complete your documentation. Don't hesitate to ask for help here. This is a new experience and you may not be able to think clearly for a while. The entire experience may leave you a bit shaken — and that's perfectly normal.

If you're still working with a preceptor, share your feelings and concerns about the code situation. If you're off orientation, you should make an opportunity to discuss your first code situation with a colleague. It will help you to review critically your role in the code situation and provide guidelines for future codes.

Speaking with family members

Usually, a doctor speaks with family members after a code situation, especially if the outcome is poor. Sometimes, however, the nurse may accompany the doctor to speak with the family and commonly stays with the family to comfort them long after the doctor has left.

Delivering bad news (or simply being present when it's delivered) is never easy. You may want to ask a more experienced nurse to sit in on your family interaction after your first code situation. There's never a "right thing to say" when people are reacting to a sudden tragedy. Sometimes, the best medicine is a listening ear and a large dose of compassion.

Nonmedical emergencies

Not all emergencies are medical emergencies. Perhaps you'll happen upon a fire or smoke. Don't panic. Use the emergency number that has been provided to you or is located on each phone. It's also helpful to keep a list of emergency phone numbers readily available.

Competencies

Competencies are the activities and skills within nursing that one must be able to perform. The facility outlines the competencies expected of the nursing staff. The facility is also expected to assess and validate competencies as a way of determining a new employee's ability to perform the expectations of her role in the facility setting.

Nursing skills

As a part of your orientation, you'll receive a checklist of skills that you must perform before the completion of your orientation. Much like the skills checklists you used in nursing school, this list is used to track skills deemed essential.

Once isn't enough!

Understand that performing a skill one time doesn't equal competency. Competency means that you can apply the knowledge along with the skill necessary to complete the task. Achieving competency also requires familiarity with facility policies and procedures. Your skills will improve, as will the time it takes to complete a skill.

Slow and steady

As a new graduate, you may be a bit disorganized and complete your assignments more slowly, but you can still provide safe, competent care. As you proceed through orientation, frequently review the checklist of skills that you must complete. It commonly takes some time, but you'll eventually complete the list. You may also be expected to review and perform certain competencies on a yearly basis.

Delegation

Most nurses, not just new graduates, have difficulty delegating tasks. The National Council of State Boards of Nursing defines delegation as *the act of transferring, to a competent individual, the authority to perform a specific nursing duty in a selected situation, while the nurse remains accountable.* This definition raises concern for most nurses. Many nurses believe, "If I'm accountable, I'd better do it myself." With the complex nature of the health care system and all that's required of a registered nurse, doing everything by yourself is next to impossible.

How and to whom?

Delegation is the key to successful patient care. Effective delegation allows registered nurses to operate more effectively. (See *How to delegate safely.*)

To effectively delegate care, there are a few things to keep in mind:
• The nurse should follow the nursing process when deciding to delegate.
• The registered nurse must first assess the patient and the situation before delegating the care to assistive personnel.
• Before delegating, the nurse must make sure that the person can perform the task; be sure to let her know what information you want to receive when she has completed the task.

It sounds simple, but you must be specific when you delegate tasks because you're ultimately accountable for the care of the assigned patients. Remember that the authority to delegate comes

How to delegate safely

To ensure that delegating is done safely and successfully, nurses must have a clear understanding of their responsibilities. Nurses must remember that, although responsibility for a task has been delegated, accountability hasn't. Nurses should receive regular updates from the person assigned the task, and must ask specific questions and evaluate the outcome.

Five "rights"

The National Council of State Boards of Nursing identifies five "rights" of delegation that must be satisfied by the delegating nurse:

Right task—The task being assigned or transferred must be within the scope of abilities and practice of the individual receiving the responsibility.

Right circumstance—The individual variables involved (patient condition, environment, caregiver training) must be appropriate for delegation.

Right person—The individual receiving the responsibility must have the legal authority to perform the task. Facility policies regarding delegation must be consistent with the law.

Right direction and communication—Instructions and expectations must be clear and understood.

Right supervision and follow-up—The delegating nurse must supervise, guide, and evaluate the performance of individuals to whom she delegates. In addition to ensuring that a particular task has been successfully carried out, the delegating nurse must also provide additional training and feedback to coworkers who function under her direction.

from each individual's state Nurse Practice Act (NPA), so you'll need to review your state's NPA.

The buck stops here!

Accountability, in this case, means that you're responsible for the action of the person to whom you delegated the tasks. Nurses are responsible for the assessment, planning, implementation, and evaluation of patient care. However, the only thing that nurses can delegate is the implementation of tasks.

The registered nurse must also provide supervision, including clear directions and expected outcomes of the tasks to be performed. She must also monitor the performance of the tasks to make sure that standards of care as well as the facility's policies and procedures are maintained. Finally, she must provide documentation of the tasks completed. Evaluation of the completed, delegated task is an important component of the delegation process. This involves evaluating the patient's response, the performance of the task or tasks, and providing feedback.

Dealing with conflict

Conflict is an inevitable part of any work environment, and you must be prepared to deal with conflict as it arises. Conflicts commonly arise from different beliefs, values, perceptions, or expectations.

Nowhere to hide

Considering the fast-paced, high-stress environments in which nurses work, a conflict could arise with a nursing colleague, doctor, family member, or member of the support staff—or even a patient. So, inevitably, you'll encounter a conflict in your work environment.

> There's no doubt about it; conflicts will occur. Fortunately, there are ways to work through and solve them—without bloodshed!

Conflict-solving strategies

There are strategies for solving conflict. However, before selecting a strategy, conflict resolution starts with a thorough assessment of the problem and determining the outcome you're seeking. While the situation is occurring, try to actively listen to the discussion; avoid the desire to respond until all the details are evident. Confrontation arises when we give in to automatic and reactive responses. Being an active listener will help you choose the right strategy. Here are five proven strategies for resolving conflict:

• *Competition* is a win-lose approach and it actually forces the conflict. Sometimes it's the only strategy that will achieve the necessary change, as in an emergency when there isn't time for disagreement or to haggle over opinions. It's an assertive, autocratic style, and it's used when other strategies have failed and someone has to take charge!

• *Accommodation* is a lose-win strategy that can be used to preserve relationships. This strategy attempts to resolve the conflict by giving in to the other person, resulting in neglecting your own needs.

• *Avoidance* is a lose-lose strategy, but it can be effective in some cases. After a heated argument or discussion, it may be wise to just move away from the situation. Although this strategy is unassertive and uncooperative and only serves to postpone the conflict, the aim is to postpone the discussion to a time when the parties involved have had an opportunity to calm down and can be more constructive in discussing the issue.

• *Compromise* is a win-lose/lose-win technique, a give-and-take style of conflict. It's best used to gain a temporary settlement and serves to satisfy each party's objectives.

• *Collaboration* is a win-win approach, and this strategy is best used to maintain objectives that are agreeable to all parties involved. This is the only conflict resolution strategy that creates a win-win situation.

Working with the team

Teamwork is essential in health care. In the health care setting, the team is composed of various health care providers and support staff, each with a vital role in the patient's care. The first team you'll work with is the staff assigned to your unit on your particular shift.

Working as a team member is integral to nursing practice. For a team to function effectively, everyone must understand and respect the roles of all team members. Depending on the patient or delivery model at your particular facility, the team members will assume different roles.

Team member roles

Make sure that you understand each person's role. The team must work together to provide optimal patient care. A designated charge nurse may be responsible for making assignments or serving as a resource person for the staff. A unit secretary or clerical assistant may be responsible for answering the telephone and general administrative work. There are registered nurses, licensed practical nurses and, perhaps, unlicensed assistive personnel. Many times during your shift, you'll need to call on your coworkers for assistance. It may be a question about a procedure or a medication, or you may need assistance with a patient.

The new kid…again!

Perhaps, the unit and shift on which you'll be working has been a team for a while. When a new person arrives on the unit, she changes the existing dynamics. Try to get to know everyone. Take advantage of break time and mealtime to get to know your coworkers. You'll be surprised how much you can learn from them. Don't segregate yourself or limit yourself to just a few people. Try to avoid gossip about the other members of your team, which can destroy team cohesion. Conflict between team members can disrupt the function of a team if you're expected to "take sides."

Stuck like glue

When you work with an effective team, you'll notice a sense of cohesion among the members. An effective team displays open communication and values each team member's contribution.

Interdisciplinary team

In addition to the nursing team, you'll be working with the multidisciplinary team, or *interdisciplinary team*. These individuals also play a role in your patient's care. Such individuals include doctors, psychologists, laboratory technicians, respiratory therapists, physical therapists, occupational therapists, social workers, dietitians, chaplains or pastoral care, biomedical technicians, pharmacists, housekeeping staff, maintenance staff, and dietary staff. The patient and his support systems are commonly also considered part of this multidisciplinary team.

If it seems crowded in here it's because everyone involved with the patient's care (including the patient) is part of the interdisciplinary team.

Stay in the loop!

It's important to remember that each member of the team has a specific task to complete. Take advantage of the individual talents of the various team members. Be sure to keep the lines of communication open, keep your feedback constructive, and be willing to accept suggestions for improvement.

Communicating effectively

As health care continues to change on a daily basis, the collegiality of the health care team remains a crucial component in the delivery of care. However, with more people involved in patient care, open and honest communication is needed.

With any communication, you have the option of being passive, assertive, or aggressive. When you don't express your thoughts or feelings, you're being *passive*. Passive behavior doesn't get rid of the problem, but commonly leads to feelings of resentment or bitterness. When you express your thoughts and beliefs in an honest and direct way and are respectful of the other person's feelings, you're behaving in an *assertive* manner. When you express your thoughts and feelings in a way that humiliates or overpowers the other person, you're acting in an *aggressive* manner.

Respect is key!

When communicating with doctors and all members of the health care team, remember to treat them with the respect they deserve; they, in turn, will treat you with respect. Know what you don't know—and appreciate what they know! Always use the truth, and speak it directly and with clarity. Don't tolerate abuse from any member of the health care team or from a patient or family member.

What about the patient?

Every patient has the right to safe, competent care. Always remember, the patient is the reason you're here; everything you do should be done with the patient as the primary focus. With all that you have to do with your new job, you may be thinking, "When will I ever have time to see my patient?"

Make rounds to your patients several times each day. It sometimes feels like you spend more time communicating *about* your patients than *with* your patients or providing direct physical care. Be sure to take advantage of the time you spend with your patients. When you're with each one, give him your full attention. Try not to appear hurried or rushed. If you only have a brief time to spend with him, let him know up front the amount of time you can spend; he'll understand.

Always remember, it doesn't take additional time to be kind, attentive, and caring. A reassuring word while taking the patient's blood pressure can sometimes make up for the quantity of time you can give.

Loving what you do

Nursing is a demanding career—intellectually, emotionally, and physically. You're going to have days when you can't remember why you chose this profession. These are the days when you've had to deal with an emergency situation, a difficult patient, or short staffing.

Don't worry, Mr. Brown. Everything will be OK.

Doing good

If, each day, you think about the positive influence you had on your patients, you'll restore your spirit. Perhaps you were able to provide intimate care to someone who was dying. Maybe you were able to relieve someone's pain. You were there to comfort a family member suffering with their loved one. You assisted in the birth of a new baby. You comforted a child in the emergency department as he received stitches. You taught someone about his newly diagnosed disease. You were there when someone came back from the operating room. You offered a family reassurance. You helped a colleague that had a difficult assignment. You were there to offer support and guidance.

Feeling proud

Professional nursing includes various roles. Nurses are teachers, counselors, caregivers, leaders, and advocates. These are incredible roles all wrapped up in one title: Registered Nurse. Try never to lose the original enthusiasm you had for your nursing career. Seek out a nurse mentor, one who can provide encouragement when you get discouraged. Seek community with other nurses who are positive role models and love what they do.

Seeking success

You've selected a career with no limits. Continue to learn. Even if you don't pursue a formal degree, stay updated. To keep your knowledge and skills up-to-date, subscribe to a professional journal, take advantage of conference time, seek professional certification in your specialty, join a professional organization, and become an active member on facility committees. These activities can only serve to enhance your professional career.

Joining forces

As a registered nurse, you join forces with 2.7 million other nurses across the United States who provide care to patients. Nursing is a respected and trusted profession. It's a privilege to be someone's nurse. Remember, nursing is bigger than one shift, one day, one week, one unit, or one agency. Nursing is a passion and a commitment to nurture the human body and spirit. It's an extraordinary profession, second to none!

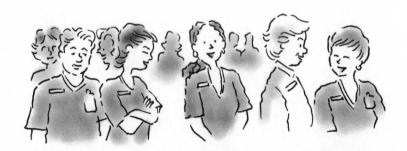

Take a break!

Interviewing tips

It's important to be prepared for the questions asked during your interview. Here are some common questions asked during interviews for nursing positions. Be prepared to answer questions similar to these before you arrive for the interview.

What's your philosophy of nursing?
_____
_____
_____
_____

What do you see yourself doing 5 years from now?
_____
_____
_____
_____

What's your greatest strength?
_____
_____
_____
_____

What's your greatest weakness?
_____
_____
_____

Tell me about a time when your course load was heavy. How did you complete all your work? When your clinical assignment was heavy, how did you manage your patient care?
_____
_____
_____
_____

Tell me about a time when you had to accomplish a task with someone who was particularly difficult to get along with.
_____
_____
_____
_____

Tell me how you handle stress.
_____
_____
_____
_____

How do you accept direction and, at the same time, maintain a critical stance regarding your ideas and values?
_____
_____
_____

Tell me how you handled an ethical dilemma (or be prepared to respond to a hypothetical ethical dilemma or clinical situation).
_____
_____
_____

Glossary

acronym: word created from the first letter or letters of each part or major parts of a compound term; used as a memory aid

acrostic: word or phrase created from the first letter of each item in a list; used as a memory aid

active listening: using planned strategies, such as taking notes or asking questions, to remember important concepts and supporting details

active reading: anticipating ideas and reading for a purpose; continually posing questions and searching for answers; used to gain a full understanding of the author's message

affirmations: repetitious, positive self-talk that usually involves simple phrases about one's capabilities

anxiety: general uneasiness, apprehension, or worry

association: process of remembering one item because of its connection to another item; linking ideas to facilitate learning

attitude: how a person approaches a task or situation; involves thoughts, feelings, and behavior

attractive distracters: incorrect options on multiple-choice tests; considered attractive because they may seem correct

behavior modification: type of external motivation involving rewards; used to divert focus from the dread of a task

Bloom's taxonomy: system developed in 1956 by Benjamin S. Bloom to describe seven levels of understanding

burnout: state that results from working too long without breaks with signs that include fatigue, boredom, and stress

closure: positive feeling that comes from completing a task, as opposed to the anxious feeling that may result from unfinished business

combination test: test that contains more than one type of question; for example, essay, multiple-choice, short-answer, or true-false questions

comprehension: understanding; using skills that include concentration, decoding, and association

comprehensive examination: examination, usually written, that tests mastery of an entire field or curriculum; test that covers all material presented since the beginning of a term

computer-assisted instruction: use of computers for instructional tasks, such as drills and practice tests

computer simulation: program that allows students to experience real-life events in the safety of a classroom

concentration: focus; ignoring distractions that may impair study habits or quality of work

concept map: approach to organizing patient data, analyzing relationships in the data, establishing patient care priorities; based upon the nursing process and displayed in a visual diagram format

cramming: an unproductive study method in which a person frantically tries to memorize a lot of information in a short period

critical pathway: documentation tool used in managed care and case management in which a time line is defined for the patient's condition and for the achievement of expected outcomes; used by caregivers to determine on any given day where the patient should be in his progress toward optimal health

critical thinking: recalling prior knowledge to translate, interpret, process, and apply new information

database: vast amounts of data organized for rapid search and retrieval (as by a computer)

esteem: assurance that one is accepted and valued; usually referring to self-esteem

flash card: card with a term or question on one side and the definition or answer on the other side; common study aid

general adaptation syndrome: theory by Hans Selye that defines the body's reaction to stress as a syndrome evolving in three stages: alarm, resistance, and exhaustion

goal: end toward which effort is directed; short- or long-term aim relating to specific, measurable outcomes

goal structure: how students relate to others who are also working toward goals; categorized as cooperative, competitive, or individualistic

graphic: illustration or visual image

intervention: nursing actions taken to meet a patient's health care needs; should reflect nurses' agreement with the patient on how to meet defined goals or expected outcomes

learning: incorporating new information; gaining knowledge; changing behavior

learning process: receiving information, gradually understanding the information, assimilating the information, and making it useful

long-term memory: ability of the brain to remember information for long periods, the duration of which directly relates to the meaningfulness of the memory; also called *semantic memory*

mantra: syllable, word, or phrase repeated again and again; used in the technique of transcendental meditation

Maslow's hierarchy: ranking of instinctual needs that human beings fill in an order from lowest to highest: physiological needs, love and belonging, self-esteem, and self-actualization

memory[1]: retention and processing of information that involves registration, working memory, short-term memory, and long-term memory; lowest level of understanding in Bloom's taxonomy

memory[2]: where a computer stores information, on the hard drive or a disk

mental pictures: most common way for the mind to process information; commonly called the *key to memorizing*

mnemonics: memory aids, such as acronyms, acrostics, associations, and rhymes

motivation: reason for doing something, which can be internal or external

National Council Licensure Examination (NCLEX): standardized examination taken by graduate nurses; passing this examination results in demonstration of minimum level knowledge of safe nursing practice and results in licensure

network: interrelated group or system; two or more linked computer systems

nursing diagnosis: clinical judgment made by a nurse about a patient's response to actual or potential health problems or life processes; describes a patient problem that the nurse can legally solve; may apply to families and communities as well as individual patients

nursing process: systematic approach to identifying a patient's problems and then taking nursing actions to address them; steps include assessing the patient's problems, forming a diagnostic statement, iden-tifying expected outcomes, creating a plan to achieve expected outcomes and solve the patient's problems, implementing the plan or assigning another to implement it, and evaluating the plan's effectiveness

noncomprehensive examination: test that covers information presented only since the last test

objective test: examination that involves choosing among provided answers; for example, multiple-choice, matching, or true-false questions

objectivity: ability to report information without personal opinion or bias

open-book examination: examination in which the student is allowed to use supplementary materials, such as notes, textbooks, charts, or crib sheets; tests a student's ability to locate and process information quickly

oral examination: examination used to measure a student's ability to analyze and integrate information as well as the ability to respond quickly in an organized manner; commonly given as a final test before awarding a degree

outlining: sequential process of organizing information according to major concepts and supporting details

overlearning: reviewing the same information several times using different study methods

overstudy: continuing to study after the point at which the material is known

paraphrase: restating main ideas and explanations rather than memorizing material word-for-word

passive note-taking: using taped or borrowed notes

plagiarism: using another person's work without citing the source; treated as stealing

postlecture reading: additional resources not covered during class that help a student focus on information emphasized in a lecture and deepen a student's understanding of the subject

practice: repetition that may involve silent rereading, rewriting, diagramming, vocalizing, or discussing information

prepared cramming: pretest review session done by a student who has been studying wisely

pretest: use of a test to evaluate baseline knowledge at a point before another test with similar content

previewing: recalling previous knowledge of a subject to create a mental outline of upcoming class information

primary sources: original documents, such as speeches or books, used in research

procrastination: putting off activities until later; letting low-priority tasks get in the way of high-priority ones

progressive relaxation: technique of gradually releasing control of each muscle from head to toe

reciprocal teaching: technique for practicing reading comprehension that involves the use of five strategies good readers use most when reading: prediction, clarification, visualization, questioning, and summarizing

recitation: orally replying to study questions; useful study technique sometimes used as a classroom exercise

registration: receiving and acknowledging new information without understanding it

regressing: constantly rereading; a habit that slows reading speed

rehearsal: repetition that may involve spaced study, previewing, recitation, study partners, or overlearning

rehearsal process: reading material, thinking about it, reciting it, answering questions, and then repeating the process

schedule: time-management tool that can be long- or short-term and should include study time

secondary sources: documents that interpret, evaluate, describe, or otherwise restate the work of primary sources

short-term memory: ability of the brain to store information briefly, which lasts only seconds or minutes unless reinforced; also called *episodic memory*

skimming: first phase of reading that involves looking at pictures, captions, headings, introductory paragraphs, and table of contents; commonly called *previewing*

social network: relationships among people in a group

social support: people who provide assistance in meeting basic needs

spaced study: alternating study sessions with breaks; very beneficial when alternating fifteen minutes of study with very short breaks; also known as *distributed practice*

spreadsheet: ledger with vertical columns and horizontal rows, usually used for numerical data; computer accounting program

SQ3R: acronym for survey, question, read, recite, and review; a classic study system

stress: the body's response to demands, which appears as worry, concern, anxiety, or nervousness and can be beneficial (eustress) or damaging (distress)

stressor: source of stress that can be almost any stimulus but usually involves a conflict

subjective test: test that requires unique answers and is used to measure recall of information and skills in organizing and expressing ideas and may include short-answer, essay, or fill-in-the-blank questions

take-home examination: essentially an open-book examination but with more time allowed; usually more difficult than in-class examinations

test anxiety: test-taking situation that causes a student to experience a mental block, which may happen even if the student knows the material well

text labeling: note-taking while reading that involves identifying relationships and summarizing information; creating a kind of index to locate information more quickly

text marking: highlighting, underlining, or otherwise marking the text while reading; taking notes in the margin

text structure: how the vocabulary and topics of a text are organized

time management: means of controlling and organizing a schedule for maximum efficiency

time planning: looking ahead to organize a schedule that may refer to 1 semester, 1 week, or 1 day

trigger words: words that provide keys to an author's message; easy-to-spot, repeatedly used terms that present themes, vocabulary, or central ideas

understanding: ability to make important connections among ideas; relating new information to existing knowledge

visual aids: elements, such as maps, charts, diagrams, photographs, and illustrations that are used to explain ideas

visualization: use of mental imagery to link objects or ideas, which may involve imagining a new solution to a problem

withdrawal: physical or psychological retreat; usually resulting from anxiety or fear; social or emotional detachment

working memory: ability of the brain to select, associate, organize, and rehearse information

Index

i refers to an illustration; t refers to a table.

i refers to an illustration; t refers to a table.

i refers to an illustration; t refers to a table.

i refers to an illustration; t refers to a table.

Master the NCLEX® exam in no time with this *Incredibly Easy CD-ROM!*

This CD-ROM offers 500 NCLEX®-style questions and answers—including alternate-format questions—organized by topic: fundamentals and medical-surgical, psychiatric and mental health, maternal-neonatal, and pediatric nursing. This bonus is just one more way in which preparing for your licensing examination has become *Incredibly Easy!*

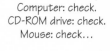

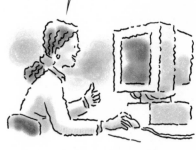

Computer: check.
CD-ROM drive: check.
Mouse: check...

Technical stuff

To operate the *Nursing Student Success Made Incredibly Easy* CD-ROM, we recommend that you have the following minimum system requirements:
- Windows 98
- Pentium 166
- 128 MB of RAM
- 10 MB of free hard-disk space
- SVGA monitor with high color (16-bit); display area set to 800 × 600
- CD-ROM drive
- mouse.

Getting started

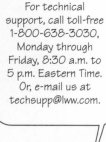

For technical support, call toll-free 1-800-638-3030, Monday through Friday, 8:30 a.m. to 5 p.m. Eastern Time. Or, e-mail us at techsupp@lww.com.

☝ Start Windows.

✌ Place the CD in your CD-ROM drive. After a few moments, the install process will automatically begin. If it doesn't, click the Start menu and select Run. Type *D:\setup.exe* (where *D:* is the letter of your CD-ROM drive) and then click OK.

🤟 Follow the on-screen installation instructions.
It's that easy!

Legal stuff

This work is protected by copyright. No part of this work may be reproduced in any form or by any means, including photocopying, or utilized by any information storage and retrieval system without written permission from the copyright owner.

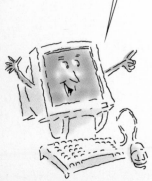